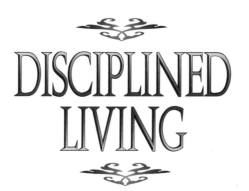

DISCIPLINED LIVING

By Boyd Luter
Looking Back, Moving On: Applying Biblical Principles of Freedom to Your Life

By Boyd Luter and Kathy McReynolds
Truthful Living: What Christianity Really Teaches about Recovery

What the New Testament

DISCIPLINED

Teaches about

LIVING

Recovery and Discipleship

BOYD LUTER

AND

KATHY McREYNOLDS

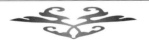

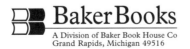
Baker Books

A Division of Baker Book House Co
Grand Rapids, Michigan 49516

Published by Baker Books
a division of Baker Book House Company
P.O. Box 6287, Grand Rapids, MI 49516-6287

Published in association with the literary agency of
Alive Communications
P.O. Box 49068
Colorado Springs, CO 80949

Printed in the United States of America

Library of Congress Cataloging-in-Publication Data

Luter, Boyd.
    Disciplined living : what the New Testament teaches about recovery and discipleship / Boyd Luter and Kathy McReynolds.
      p. cm.
    Includes bibliographical references and indexes.
    ISBN 0-8010-5243-2 (pbk.)
    1. Bible. N.T.—Criticism, interpretation, etc. 2. Christian life—Biblical teaching. 3. Rehabilitation—Biblical teaching. 4. Mental health—Biblical teaching. I. McReynolds, Kathy, 1960–. II. Title.
BS2545.C48L88 1995
261.8'3229—dc20   95-23624

Contents

Preface

$\mathbb{B}$etween the two of us, this is the fourth bold step we have attempted to further the integration of psychology and theology (in the broader sense of the word) from the, until very recently, overlooked biblical side of the mix. Both of us contributed in different ways to the *Life Recovery Bible* (Tyndale, 1992), which sought to give an introductory biblical basis to the recovery counseling framework that had virtually overwhelmed the evangelical counseling arena, beginning in the later 1980s. Boyd then wrote *Looking Back, Moving On: Applying Biblical Principles of Freedom to Your Life* (Navpress, 1993) as a more in-depth scriptural exposition of what a truly biblical approach to recovery looks like. Following that, we collaborated on *Truthful Living: What Christianity Really Teaches about Recovery* (Baker, 1994), the first systematic theological critique of the emerging evangelical recovery viewpoint and movement.

Disciplined Living fits hand-in-glove with *Truthful Living* from a methodology standpoint. It is a New Testament theology, meaning that it traces the thought patterns of each of the individual New Testament writers. Sometimes, as in the case of Paul's letters, we break things down book by book—in a way similar to the outlook of the brand-new *New Testament Theology* series, edited by James D. G. Dunn (T & T Clark). This volume thus fills the methodology gap in our "paper trail" between basic exegesis/application and systematic theology.

Yet there is much more that is groundbreaking about *Disciplined Living*. The subject matter of this book is not just recovery. It is a comprehensive weaving together of recovery and discipleship. In that sense, it is our attempt to ask and answer, where should the parallel transformation/growth processes of recovery and discipleship take you over the longhaul? As will be seen, and in strong agreement with what we learned in writing *Truthful Living,* Christlikeness is the answer for both biblically rooted recovery and discipleship.

Further, there is a consistent utilization of literary analysis in *Disciplined Living,* probing the structure of many New Testament passages or whole books for fresh insights that are helpful in understanding New Testament teaching on recovery and discipleship. It is our conviction that scholarly angles, such as literary structural patterns, can be mined for nuggets that have great practical applications, and we have attempted to do so.

After all, if the original writers employed certain kinds of flourishes in writing style to strengthen, make more colorful, and clarify, aren't we being shortchanged if we don't understand the intent of these flourishes? Even if such features are notably different from the way people write today, can we afford to impoverish our understanding and grounds of application by shrugging our shoulders and ignoring the distinctive (often elegant) communication formats of other cultures? Our answers to questions like these, mixed with passion for the subject matter, fueled our study and shaped our presentation of *Disciplined Living.*

Our heartfelt appreciation is due to:

Our families, for Spirit-empowered patience (Gal. 5:22) with our deadline-driven writing schedules.

Allan Fisher and Mary Suggs of Baker Book House, for the gracious opportunity to develop the creative slant of this material in book form, with its significant implications for both the scholarly and practical realms.

Talbot School of Theology, Biola University, for the opportunity to ground a considerable amount of the thinking re-

flected here, on both recovery and discipleship, in the inter-
active classroom setting.

Greg Johnson and Rick Christian of Alive Communications,
for working out the details so that we could concentrate on
research and writing.

All who encouraged us that what we were doing is needed; and
all who questioned and challenged us to think deeper, wider,
and better.

Introduction

A Timely Warning

There can be little doubt that Jude was a wise veteran disciple. Even if he was not converted to faith in Jesus Christ until after the resurrection, as seems likely (Matt. 13:55–57; John 7:5; Acts 1:14),[1] Jude would have been a disciple in the most basic sense of "learner, follower"[2] for about thirty years or more by the time he wrote the New Testament letter that carries his name.[3] Further, his self-description of "bond-servant" (Jude 1) carries with it the implication of voluntary commitment, befitting Christ's disciple (Luke 14:26–33).

In a very real sense, though, it can also be said that Jude well understood biblical recovery.[4] Though that specific term is not found in the New Testament, the family background in which Jude grew up appears to have been a breeding ground for at least (what would be called today) moderate recovery issues.[5]

For example, the fact that Jesus, as the oldest child, was brilliant and perfect in his behavior (literally!) would have naturally spawned significant sibling rivalry and resentment. If Joseph and Mary fell prey to the temptation to make comparisons or to set their standards for the other children too high because of Jesus, the likelihood of perfectionism is considerable. Further, since there is no mention of Joseph after Jesus was twelve years old (Luke

13

2:42–48), there is a significant possibility that the family was bereaved of the father while the younger children, like Jude, were still at a formative stage[6]—an even more traumatic loss in a patriarchal society.

Add to that the sense of abandonment that Jude may well have felt when Jesus went off to public ministry at about age thirty (Luke 3:23), leaving the support of the family, including their widowed mother, Mary, on the shoulders of the younger brothers, including Jude. Then there would have been the mixed feelings over Jesus' miracles and strange teachings, such as the redefining of family in terms of spiritual and discipleship relationships (Matt. 12:46–50). Finally, there was the anguish of Jesus being executed by the Roman soldiers and Jewish teachers (Matt. 27:35–50), even as their mother looked on (27:55–56).

Thus, in effect, Jude also began a substantial (biblical) recovery reorientation at the time of his conversion, along with beginning the process of discipleship. In that regard, he can be rightly considered a reliable guide in both arenas. We do well to hear his insights and heed his warnings![7]

Sadly, seldom have Jude's insights and warnings been heeded less than by the evangelical Recovery Movement in the United States, and the evangelical churches with which it is loosely aligned, in the mid-1990s. This book will focus on the diagnosis and treatment offered by Jude as well as all the other New Testament writers. It will utilize an adapted biblical theology approach that will balance the systematic theology methodology of our recent book, *Truthful Living: What Christianity Really Teaches about Recovery*.[8] Approaching the issues that have developed within American evangelicalism in the late twentieth century through the lens of New Testament theology will allow the paralleling of circumstances and problems, which are strikingly similar at point after point.

That the introductory set of such parallels was chosen to come from Jude carries with it a touch of irony for us. It was noted in the preface of *Truthful Living* that we felt compelled to change directions even as we conceived that project, much as Jude had in regard to his letter (v. 3). In that book, we sought to provide a previously undeveloped perspective on recovery, anchoring it at every point to "the faith which was once for all delivered to the saints" (Jude 3).

In the less than a year and a half since that manuscript was completed, things have changed considerably in terms of the mood of the dialogue between some of the leading evangelical recovery thinkers and writers on the one hand and the wider evangelical sector on the other. The virtually unprecedented success of the recovery programs and publications from the later 1980s through 1992 has stirred up a very strong negative reaction in many quarters.[9]

Unfortunately, as often happens when passions run hot on a subject, further polarization has taken place. Accordingly, the two most visible (or, at least, vocal!) present positions on evangelical recovery and psychology are what I term "throwing the baby out with the bathwater" and "buying it hook, line, and sinker."[10] The one side has become even more heated in its across-the-board antipsychology rhetoric, while the other side has defensively gone further in the opposite direction, championing positions in too many cases that have less and less valid biblical theological moorings.[11]

As we have written in earlier publications, we continue to believe that both of these opposite positions represent extremes. The balanced position is found between the two, by rigorously critiquing the findings of psychology, in regard to the diagnosis and treatment of emotional problems, through a full-orbed biblical grid that rests squarely on the bedrock-evangelical tenet that the Bible is the final authority in all matters related to faith and practice.[12]

Appeal to those holding both polar positions must, in many ways, be quite different because their assumptions and starting points are so far apart. However, in one sense, because both groups are comprised of self-professed evangelicals, a similar appeal is possible. If they believe the Bible, they will listen when the question is: What do the Scriptures say?

That is what this book is intended to be and do: less what Luter and McReynolds think; more what Luke, Matthew, and all the other inspired New Testament writers (2 Tim. 3:16) have to say on matters presently troubling the evangelical church. So, on to their timeless (i.e., in this case, speaking very directly to the timely questions and needs that are the focus of the current debate) insights.

As stated earlier, Jude is first in line. The problem that had focused Jude's wise resolve (Jude 3) to address his Christian readers (v. 1) was the subtle intrusion of certain persons who had gone overboard in regard to the concept of grace. This view of grace taken to the extreme had resulted in licentious behavior and an effective denial of Jesus Christ, whom Jude describes as "our only Master and Lord" (v. 4).

While it is certainly possible that the error that Jude is sketching out in verse 4 is of a foundational doctrinal variety, it seems more likely that the heresy is at least primarily moral-behavioral.[13] That means that there must not have been any overt theological defection involved, hence the ability of such people to have "crept in unnoticed" (v. 4).

The bulk of Jude's letter is given over to showing how the Scripture (and one extrabiblical source[14]) consistently condemns such ungodly behavior (vv. 5–18). Further, it accuses the troublemakers of being "worldly-minded" and without the Holy Spirit (v. 19).

Such descriptions are highly ironic when comparison is made to the present dispute over recovery in American evangelicalism, for example. Though we are not aware that the term *ungodly* has been thrown around, muttering about moral-behavioral looseness is often heard in hushed tones, in which the code word *grace* is used to paper over everything from unconfessed bitterness to occasional gross lapses in sexual behavior or substance abuse.

Also, while there is obviously no direct connection of any sort, the Greek term *psychikos* (translated "worldly-minded") is a kindred term to *psychē*, from which the English term *psychology* is derived. Since those who are highly suspicious of the use of psychology by evangelicals are frequently convinced that psychologists and counselors are under the spell of a secular (i.e., worldly) discipline, it behooves those in psychology roles to make it abundantly clear that such is not the case by avoiding as much as possible even the implication of being out of bounds (1 Thess. 5:22).[15]

It does no one any good to bristle against criticism and claim the right to do your own thing. Spiritual profit, edification, and a good testimony for the Lord comes from living within the boundaries of biblical behavioral standards (1 Cor. 10:23). To do otherwise is to engage in a kind of denial that is at least as serious as the commonly referred to psychological variety: denying the only Master and Lord, Jesus Christ, by using grace as an excuse for controversial, licentious behavior (Jude 4).

A final serious concern of Jude, which is sometimes true of those on the psychological side of the aisle in the current debate, is the lack of the Holy Spirit in the lives of those Jude is opposing (v. 19). This is in no way to judge whether the "fruit of the Spirit" (Gal. 5:22–23) or the filling of the Spirit (Eph. 5:18) is present in a certain evangelical counselor's or psychologist's life. It is, however, tragic to observe how appallingly little about the Holy Spirit is found in the psychologically based writings that dominated the early recovery boom in evangelical circles[16] and has been only minimally corrected since.

So, there is Jude's piercing diagnosis of the subtle problem that had to be corrected in the first century church! But what is the treatment he prescribes that believers then and now must take to heart?

1. They need to actively build themselves up in the faith (i.e., the Scriptures and their theological teaching)[17] and pray in the power of the Holy Spirit (Jude 20). Those directions will certainly please those distrustful of psychology!
2. They are to emphasize the "love of God" and the "mercy of our Lord Jesus Christ" (v. 21). That will undoubtedly appeal to the psychologists and counselors!
3. Jude states, however, that his readers must deal with others in the application of mercy (vv. 22–23) in various ways. Some need a very sensitive approach (v. 22); some need a much more directive one (v. 23a). But in cases related to morality, *always* be careful for your own spiritual life and testimony (v. 23b)![18] That will cut *both* ways!

There it is: a simple (but not easy!) and balanced approach to correct subtle grace-become-license problems troubling the water of the church in any generation. But what does this accomplish long-term?

A lot for eternity, if you're in it for the long haul! After all, as the much-more-than-a-mere-doxology in Jude 24–25 proclaims, the Lord is fully able to keep those in recovery from stumbling (v. 24a) throughout this life. Also, he provides the dynamic for the kind of committed discipleship that will make for great joy when you stand before the Lord (v. 24b) and glorify, not deny (v. 4), Jesus Christ.

It is our hope that those who read these pages will sense our concern for those who are "beloved" of the Lord (Jude 1) and us (v. 3) on both sides of the aisle, as well as our desire to cling to his Word first, while carefully utilizing the biblically and theologically legitimate insights of the evangelical psychological community. The bottom line, though, must always be to glorify our Lord in all that we write and do in connection with those in emotional pain (vv. 4, 25)!

Soli Deo Gloria!

Note to the reader: The authors have each written chapters on the New Testament books for which they have expertise. Please refer to the top of each left-hand page for the author of a particular chapter.

1

Discipleship or Denial?

Gospel of Matthew

It is a very common thing for the Gospel of Matthew to be viewed as a "manual for discipleship."[1] That is quite understandable. After all, the First Gospel is crowned by the risen Lord's command: "Go therefore and make disciples of all the nations" (Matt. 28:19). Also, there is a strong emphasis on the training of the twelve disciples that were closest to Jesus (e.g., Matt. 10:1–4).

There is, however, much more to the Gospel of Matthew than discipleship (though not less!). For example, much of the biblical basis of the well-known Twelve Steps of Recovery is understood to have come from Matthew. Those ideas were generalized (i.e., chapter and verse were deleted) for the widest possible practical impact. [2]

Thus, much about recovery could be discussed in regard to the Gospel of Matthew. Particularly, Matthew has much to say about denial—a very important recovery concept. The best known instance of denial in Matthew, of course, is the apostle Peter's threefold denial of knowing Jesus Christ after his arrest in the Garden of Gethsemane (Matt. 26:31–35, 58–75).

Peter's denial, however, is only the tip of the iceberg. As will be seen, the concept of denial fairly frequently intersects the concept of discipleship in Matthew, even as it clearly did with Peter (in the instance just cited).

In this foundational chapter of this book, I will survey the extensive teaching on denial that can be gleaned from Matthew as well as provide an overview of its even more extensive content related to discipleship. There are various points at which the material in both areas crosses paths, and I will develop two of these in particular.

Key Definitions

The basic meaning of the term normally translated "disciple" (Greek *mathetes*) is "learner, pupil, or follower."[3] Thus, in general, discipleship is the process of being a pupil or follower of a particular teacher (or viewpoint).

Within the scope of becoming a Christian and growing spiritually as a believer, however, *discipleship* in regard to Jesus Christ must be more closely defined. That is true if for no other reason than that Christ demands the highest level of commitment from the person who would be his disciple (Luke 14:26–33; Matt. 10:24–39).

Thus, biblical discipleship may be defined as "the process of learning about Jesus and how to follow him as a committed lifestyle." Still, such a definition does not fully reflect the about-face that is necessary from the pre-Christian pattern of life.

This is a point at which the reality of a biblical theology of recovery comes very much into play. Since the human heart is, naturally, "more deceitful than all else and is desperately sick" (Jer. 17:9), salvation and discipleship are far more than a simple continuation, or even a minor adjustment, from life outside of Christ.

So, tempered by theological and behavioral reality, it is better to define discipleship as the process of *re*learning about Jesus or *re*directing your life to follow Jesus as a life pattern. In that sense, it is no coincidence that *re*covery also starts with the same prefix (*re*). Both are about a substantial change of direction of your life.[4]

In this light, denial is seen to be a major roadblock on the path of discipleship. This can be quickly surmised from a general definition of *denial:* "The persistent unwillingness to view and face circumstances and/or people as they realistically exist."

In the case of discipleship, that unrecognized reality would include who Jesus Christ is and his claim on a person's life. One level of denial keeps a person from becoming a Christian. Another level of denial can cause a person to break down on, or veer from, the narrow pathway (Matt. 7:13–14; Luke 13:24) of discipleship. Both levels will be seen in the survey of denial in the Gospel of Matthew. First, I will briefly discuss the writer and likely circumstances behind the Gospel in order to probe his interest in denial and discipleship.

The Life (Change!) and Time of Matthew

The First Gospel is, technically, an anonymous document, as are the other three Gospels. There is, however, a very strong likelihood that it was written by Matthew, the apostle and former tax collector (Matt. 9:9; 10:3).[5] If Matthew was not the author, it is fair to say that there is no strong alternate candidate.

What is known about Matthew certainly qualifies him to author such an account that emphasizes both denial and discipleship. For example, in order to take on a role as hated by his fellow Jews and as corrupt as being a Roman tax collector, Matthew (a.k.a. "Levi," in Mark 2:14–17 and Luke 5:27–29) certainly had to be in denial to some degree. On the other hand, leaving his role as tax collector to follow Jesus as a disciple (Matt. 9:9) represented a massive change in the direction of life and corresponding commitment.[6]

Fortunately, the Gospel of Matthew virtually telegraphs both who its intended original readers were as well as what Matthew's purpose was in addressing them. The impressive number of Old Testament quotes, paraphrases, and echoes make it almost certain that the first readers of the First Gospel were Jews. Also, though the first verse of the book indicates that it was intended to prove and explain that Jesus was the rightful king of Israel (Matt. 1:1), the following family tree strongly implies that the initial reference to Jesus as "the son of Abraham" was equally significant.

In Genesis 12:3 it had been promised to Abraham that, in some sense, "all the families of the earth shall be blessed" through his descendants (12:2). Balancing the Great Commission's scope of discipling "all the nations" (Matt. 28:19), which is found at the conclusion of Matthew, is a similar, but more subtle, emphasis at the beginning. Unexpectedly, four Gentile women—Tamar (Matt. 1:3), Rahab (1:5), Ruth (1:5), and Bathsheba ("her who had been the wife of Uriah," 1:6)—are included in Jesus' messianic genealogy.[7] These names indicate that the Lord had, in fact, included the Gentiles in his plan of redemption from the beginning!

Thus, given the typical Jewish viewpoint of the day (i.e., that Gentiles were "dogs"; see Matt. 15:26–27), Matthew was also taking on the nationwide denial of the Jews in regard to the Gentiles also having a place in God's plan. Like the Jews, the Gentiles needed bottom-line eternal recovery (i.e., new life in Christ) and the commitment of discipleship.

The most slippery of the background issues related to Matthew's Gospel is its dating.[8] The fact that Matthew is placed first among the four Gospels is largely due to the widespread belief that it was written first, perhaps as early as the late 40s of the first century. Other evangelicals believe that it could have been written in the 50s or 60s, some as late as around A.D. 70. There is nothing close to a current consensus.

Interestingly, though I think that the earlier date is slightly more likely, either of the polar possibilities would be of significance for this study. A late 40s date would be close in time to the Jerusalem council in Acts 15, which dealt directly with what was involved in Gentiles becoming Christians. A date around A.D. 70 would be near the time of the destruction of Jerusalem by the Romans.

Either point of origin would have been emotionally traumatic for most Jews who read the Gospel of Matthew. There would have been a strong tendency to remain in denial in regard to both accepting Gentiles as spiritual equals and to facing the shattering of the Jewish capital and temple.

From a discipleship perspective, again both dates would seem to have merit. The late 40s date would coincide with the fleshing out of Christ's command to "make disciples of all the nations" (Matt. 28:19) in Paul's first missionary journey (Acts 13–14). An A.D. 70 dating would imply that the Gospel and the Great Commission must necessarily go on beyond the destruction of the temple to the end of the age (Matt. 24:2, 14; 28:19–20).[9]

The Shape of Denial in Matthew's Gospel

When looking at denial from a counseling standpoint, it is most commonly seen in regard to painful losses or some other change in status. To one degree or another, the person in question can't face it or can't handle it and is, thus, in denial.[10]

However, it is not at all implausible that denial can be a chronic state. For example, I was most certainly hunkered down in an emotional turtle shell of denial in two wide-ranging areas when struck down by viral pneumonia in 1991. First, there was ongoing denial about a painful son-to-father relationship. Second, there was denial about personal limitations. Both contributed mightily to my crashing and burning physically and emotionally.[11]

Allow me to explain a little further, because both kinds of my denial are roughly parallel to the kinds of denial that are reflected in the Gospel of Matthew. In the first case, my anger and frustration did not allow me to see either my father or myself in a realistic light. In the second case, my unwillingness to face my inability to summon the strength and answers to my problems set me up for a major physical burnout.

The twin focus of most of the denial in Matthew is also seen to be a life-defining relationship and personal limitations but with even more on the line than in my case. Over and over, denial is related to issues of proper relationship with the life-giving Lord. (Note especially the alarming wording of Matt. 10:33!)

Specifically, the Jews whom Matthew was both writing about and writing to did not see Jesus Christ for who he really is. As a result of that deficiency by denial, they could not see themselves realistically. Why? Because human sinfulness and inability to pull off our own salvation is most clearly seen in the light of the true understanding of the person of Jesus, the sinless God-man.

Now we are in position to rapidly survey how Matthew presents Jesus as seen through the eyes of denial. You will see that each of the examples contains an element of truth. However, for the balanced, disciplined living that is the essence of both biblical recovery and discipleship to take place, you must face up to the truth, the *whole* truth, and nothing but the truth.

1. *Jesus was shortsightedly viewed by certain powerful figures as merely a rival for power.* For example, that seems to have been the case with Herod the Great. Matthew 2:1–18 portrays Herod's jealous attempt to kill the infant Jesus. It is also insightful to notice that Herod's quest was set in motion by the question of the Magi: "Where is He who has been born King of the Jews?" (Matt. 2:2).

Two other classic examples are found in Matthew of a deep-seated unwillingness to see Jesus as anything beyond a pretender to the throne. Satan's approach was to tempt Jesus in the wilderness (Matt. 4:1–11), climaxing in the offer of power to be bestowed by Satan if Jesus would worship him (4:8–10). The other example is the various Jewish and Roman leaders, whose trumped-up arrest of Jesus, illegal kangaroo court trial, and crucifixion of the sinless Lord (Matt. 26–27) revolved around the question, "Are You the King of the Jews?" (27:11; see also 27:37).

2. *Many people saw Jesus Christ as only a great teacher.* During the Sermon on the Mount (Matt. 5–7), the unbelieving multitudes apparently rejoined the disciples (5:1; 7:28–29). This mass of people was clearly amazed at Jesus' authoritative teaching, but there is no indication at this point that they saw Jesus as the Messiah-Savior.

Further, in Jesus' hometown of Nazareth, the populace was "astonished" (Matt. 13:54) at his teaching in the local synagogue. However, they did not seek to understand Jesus beyond asking, "Is this not the carpenter's son?" (v. 55).[12]

3. *It was quite common for Jesus to be perceived as only a great miracle worker.* The people in Nazareth were also drawn to his miracles (Matt. 13:54), but nothing more. So were most of those in Chorazin, Bethsaida, and Capernaum, who did not change their perspective at all about Jesus (11:20–24). As best as we can tell, that was the viewpoint of the vast majority of those present for the miraculous feeding of the five thousand (14:13–21) and the later feeding of the four thousand (15:32–39).

4. *It is clear that Jesus was frequently taken to be only a great prophet.* That was apparently the overwhelming understanding of the crowds lining the road at the triumphal entry (21:11). That defi-

cient understanding is best seen in Peter's answer to Jesus' question: "Who do people say that the Son of Man is?" (Matt. 16:13). The options ranged from John the Baptist to Elijah to Jeremiah or another prophet (v. 14). The key point here, though, is that the multiple-choice options on who Jesus was *all* limited him to prophet status!

5. *Often Jesus was reduced to "Messiah as you understand him."* For Christians reading this book, this final angle on denial seen in the Gospel of Matthew is the most likely to be seen in your own experience or that of your fellow believers. It also parallels a troubling deficiency of much of the evangelical Recovery Movement.

Peter fell prey to this kind of denial *long* before he denied Jesus three times on the night before the crucifixion. Peter flatly denied that Jesus' suffering, death, and resurrection in Jerusalem would take place (Matt. 16:21–22). Peter apparently held a tenacious stereotype of Jesus' role as Messiah. He had no trouble accepting Jesus as the divine Messiah (16:16), but he refused to face the whole Jesus, or at least his whole mission.

Jesus' response to Peter is very significant for application of a biblical recovery perspective. The Lord rebuked Peter, saying, in effect, that his limited view was both satanically inspired and man-centered (or self-centered; 16:23), though Peter apparently hadn't noticed that either was the case.

Lest the point be missed, a parallel deficiency is present with the Twelve Steps program's "God as you understand him" perspective. If the apostle Peter was rebuked for his well-intentioned but shortsighted outlook (16:21–23), would it not be true that the Lord would similarly rebuke attempts to define him in our terms today? Is it too much to conclude that an emotions-based versus scripturally based understanding of Jesus (or God) today is still, ultimately, satanic and egotistical, even if the person is unaware of what shaped the viewpoint?

This rapid-fire study of denial in Matthew's Gospel can also open the eyes of the reader to a vitally important principle that bridges between recovery and discipleship. In a very real sense, you are in denial whenever you refuse to see Jesus for who he really is (i.e., the whole package of his person and work). Obviously, if a person is locked into denial, he or she cannot progress very far in recovery.

Similarly, a deficient view of Christ makes for a distorted discipleship. Faulty understanding breeds faulty commitment. Thus, progress on the discipleship front essentially grinds to a halt also.

So, until "God as you understand him" is replaced by "God as Scripture presents him," there is the ever-lurking danger that the content and direction of the recovery process is somehow, behind the scenes, being shaped by Satan and the human ego. The same is essentially true of a pick-and-choose "Jesus as you understand him" approach to discipleship.

A Look at Recovery-Related Discipleship in Matthew

When you approach the Gospel of Matthew on the subject of discipleship, there is a treasure of material to investigate. There also is a wealth of excellent published material to enhance your study of disciples and discipleship in Matthew.[13]

Matthew's depiction of following Christ as a disciple involves much that also has implications in regard to recovery. The First Gospel's extensive development of discipleship includes at least the following twelve points:

1. *Following Christ involves turning from your natural lifestyle to a supernaturally remolded life*. Of course, this is seen vividly in the life of Matthew, the former tax collector. However, the principle is focused most clearly in regard to the call to discipleship of Simon Peter, Andrew, James, and John (Matt. 4:18–22).[14]

In calling these four fishermen to follow him (vv. 19, 21), Jesus promised to make them "fishers of men." Now, that does not mean that they never went out in a boat in search of fish again. In fact, in two cases it seems that a return to fishing taught these key disciples crucial lessons (see Luke 5:4–11; John 21:3–8). It does mean, though, that having learned the principles and process of effective fishing well, they were to now apply their energies and insight to the new, supernatural task of evangelizing humankind.

Isn't it amazing how the Lord never wastes anything in the background of a disciple? No matter what you were (or did) before you trusted the Lord Jesus and began to follow him, he will graciously use what you learned from your old life to enhance your growth, as well as the salvation and growth of others!

It is fair to say that the Lord's agelong discipling program (Matt. 28:19–20) is by far the largest job-retraining program in all of history. One of the reasons that it has had such staying power is that it so frequently builds on previously honed natural abilities in sharpening new supernatural gifts and skills. This ties in well with balanced biblical recovery, which seeks to anchor the transformation of recovery in God's supernatural power, present in the believer's life.

2. *As Christ's disciple, you make him the foundation of your life in order to be prepared for the storms of life.* The passage that crowns Jesus' Sermon on the Mount makes this point with force.

Hard on the heels of Jesus' memorable analogies of the two gates (Matt. 7:13–14) and two kinds of trees and fruit (vv. 16–20) as two opposite ways of conducting one's life comes his illustration of the wise and foolish house builders (vv. 24–27). All three of these word pictures, especially the last, clearly indicate that his disciples, whom he is seeking to teach (Matt. 5:1), must make a foundational choice to hear and apply Jesus' words (v. 24). That same point applies in recovery: Without understanding hand-in-hand with action, there is no recovery!

3. *A follower of Christ becomes sensitive to the spiritual harvest and open to becoming a harvester.* Matthew 9:36 reflects Jesus' intense compassion for the dejected, leaderless masses to whom he ministered. Then the Savior sought to impress the spiritual neediness of the multitudes on his closest disciples, using the figure of a harvest (vv. 37–38).

The pressing problem that Jesus addresses is the lack of workers available to bring in the spiritual bumper crop (9:37). As well as enlisting their prayers for such harvesters to be provided (v. 38), Christ seems to be strongly implying that "His disciples" (v. 37) should consider becoming harvest workers themselves.

Certainly at least some of the disciples who heard Jesus speak of the harvest that day were later involved in the evangelistic ministry of the early church seen in the Book of Acts. As a partial answer to the prayer Jesus asked his disciples to pray, they harvested an amazing crop of new disciples in Jerusalem, Judea, and

Samaria, and throughout the known world of the day (Acts 1:8). (Excuse the pun, but I wonder if the agricultural machinery manufacturer didn't rip off "International Harvester" from Jesus.) Relatedly, should not disciples who work through discipleship issues desire to help the spiritual "harvest" of those around them who also desperately need recovery?

4. *As a disciple of Christ, you work together with other disciples you wouldn't naturally get along with to accomplish Christ's mission.* This is seen in the passage that immediately follows Jesus' words about the evangelistic harvest that was just discussed.

Matthew 10:1–6 records the commissioning for ministry of Jesus' twelve closest disciples, whom he chose to send out as apostles. The mission that they were to carry out would have been a great challenge under the most ideal circumstances and with the best, most compatible, relationships.

Unfortunately, in the middle of the listing of the Twelve, the reader encounters two individuals who make "the Odd Couple" seem well matched by comparison: Matthew, the former Roman-employed tax collector (10:3) and Simon the Zealot, a former member of an extreme Jewish nationalist sect who hated the Romans (10:4). From a political standpoint, their backgrounds faced off these two disciples-become-apostles much like Michael Kinsley and Patrick Buchanan on CNN's *Crossfire*.

Matthew seems to record this natural enmity in order to show that oil and water can indeed mix—*spiritually!* In spite of their virtually diametrically opposed backgrounds, it appears that Matthew and Simon were able to work together as disciples of Christ. Perhaps nothing else but all-out commitment to the Lord Jesus could cause two such different people to bury the hatchet, then or now. Perhaps nothing but such full-blown commitment could empower the emotional recovery from anger and distrust seen in Matthew and Simon.

In preparing to send out the Twelve to minister with authority (Matt. 10:1), Jesus instructed them at some length about the nature of worthy discipleship (see 10:37–38). In fact, the next five principles involved in following Christ (numbers five through nine) all emerge from his message to the Twelve recorded in Matthew 10.

5. *Disciples must be shrewd about the ways of the world but completely innocent of its sins.* In one sense, Jesus says, his disciples are "sheep in the midst of wolves" (Matt. 10:16). They could easily be preyed upon by the savage world around them. It would be their shrewd perceptiveness that would keep them from being eaten alive by the hostile world system. At the same time, they must constantly be careful to keep their testimonies spotless from a moral and ethical standpoint.

Sadly, this kind of balance sounds to many disciples like it comes from the dark side of the moon. The only context in which they have ever heard the term *shrewd* used has to do with marginal, if not highly questionable, practices. Thus, since they assume shrewdness is always out of bounds, they often end up being taken advantage of because of being naive and gullible.

Fortunately, Jesus' statement in Matthew 10:16 reminds disciples that shrewdness is not sinful in and of itself (see also Luke 16:8). Rather, it must be effectively paired with a moral and ethical lifestyle that is above reproach (i.e., "innocent as doves") if it is to keep from sinking into the sewer of the kind of shrewdness that is so habitually the pattern of the unsaved world and, unfortunately, the model that many people dealing with recovery issues have seen consistently in their lives.

6. *As a follower of Christ, you grow more and more into the image of your ultimate Mentor/Master.* In two proverblike assertions, Matthew 10:24–25 indicates that a disciple is to grow into the likeness of the teacher and a slave (or servant) into that of the master (Greek *kurios*, frequently translated "lord"). Since believers in Jesus Christ are both his disciples and servants, the need for simultaneous growth in learning and servanthood is crucial.

Fortunately, the Lord is on record as doing more than his share in making Christians into Christ's image (Rom. 8:28–29). The remaining question has to do with what extent we are cooperating with that process, especially when it is unpopular or painful to do so.[15] Both trusting the sovereignty of God in your life and acting on your own personal responsibility are, of course, also absolutely critical in the process of biblical recovery.

7. *You must confess your relationship with Christ openly before other people (Matt. 10:32)*. Christ only asks his disciple to do what he will do on that disciple's behalf before the heavenly Father!

The attached converse about denying Jesus is very sobering, however. Verse 33 indicates that the action of earthly denial (before men) triggers the reaction of heavenly denial (before God the Father). If nothing else that Matthew has to say about denial registers, let this sink in! Denial can produce disastrous eternal fruit! That fearful reality must be ever before the eyes of those in recovery, who might tend to slide back into denial, even ever so subtly.

8. *Make the lordship of Christ the priority relationship in your life (Matt. 10:34–37)*. In parallel to the greatest commandment in the Law (Matt. 22:36–38), to be a worthy disciple of Jesus, it is necessary to strive to love him more than your physical parents or children (10:37), no matter how much you love them!

This would have been a particularly challenging aspect of discipleship for Mary, Jesus' mother. But she definitely came to the point of loving Jesus as Lord first, then as her son, as is seen in her being described as one of the women disciples at the foot of the cross and the following events (Matt. 27:56, 61; 28:1, 5).[16] In parallel, the lordship of Christ must provide the anchoring relationship in the life of the person in recovery. This is a solid base for dealing with what are often very unhealthy relationships in the recovering individual's life.

9. *Trade your old life for the pain, humiliation, and transformation of the cross*. Matthew 10:38 makes it clear that Christ's disciple must accept much the same kind of horribly painful embarrassment that was involved in death by crucifixion in the ancient world. It would be through death—perhaps an excruciating death—to the present natural lifestyle that new, supernatural life would be gained (v. 39). It is not mere coincidence that at least the beginning and early stages of recovery are as painful (in a different, positive way) as were the previous distorted lifestyle and relationships.

10. *Become a serving disciple on the way to (possibly) becoming a servant-leader*. James and John and their mother attempted to secure the positions of honor in Jesus' coming kingdom (Matt. 20:20–21). After rebuking their lack of perspective (vv. 22–23),

Jesus spoke to the misunderstanding of true spiritual leadership by all of his disciples.

Instead of worldly power, which lords it over people (v. 25), discipleship-leadership serves others, putting them and their needs first (vv. 26–27). That is the road to effective spiritual leadership— a road Jesus himself has taken before you (v. 28)!

This balance can be achieved by a person in recovery also. The key is seeking to bring his or her self-image into conformity with Christ's image, instead of attempting to diminish self-doubt through leadership or groveling as a servant.

11. *Stand firm for Christ at life's low points, which may include substantial suffering.* Suffering and death can be highly disillusioning. Yet, it is in those Death Valleys of life that we often find out what we're really committed to, what has staying power in our lives.

Many women who followed Jesus as disciples were seen at the foot of the cross (Matt. 27:55–56), at Jesus' Death Valley, so to speak. The apostles were not there (except for John, probably; John 19:26), nor were other disciples who had been shattered by grief and disillusionment. But the women's discipleship won out over disillusionment![17] Similarly, those in recovery can anticipate seasons of disillusionment. They cannot cave into their fears at such points, however. Their faith in Christ and in the power of the Holy Spirit is indispensable for their progress and growth.

12. *Multiply yourself as a part of Christ's global disciple-making strategy.* Jesus predicted that the gospel would "be preached in the whole world for a witness to all the nations" before the end would come (Matt. 24:14). Then, he commanded all his disciples to be involved in the process of not just evangelizing, but making other disciples from among all the nations (Matt. 28:19–20).

This was to be done by a three-step process:

1. *Going* with the gospel (v. 19).
2. *Baptizing* the converts (v. 19).
3. *Teaching* them to respond with full obedience to the Lord (v. 20).

This is the process that will be seen in the Book of Acts as the Great Commission begins to be fulfilled to the ends of the earth (Acts 1:8).[18]

A Two-Way Intersection

As we conclude this foundational chapter on Matthew's teaching in regard to recovery and discipleship, obviously there is much to take in and apply on both fronts. However, before closing, it is critical to point out that, at the intersection of Recovery Road and Discipleship Way near the end of the Gospel of Matthew, there remains some overarching good news and some far-reaching bad news.

We'll get the bad news out of the way first: Matthew soberly reflects that *denial can easily undercut discipleship*. That point is emphasized in one-two-three fashion in Matthew 26–27.

1. The eleven remaining apostles broke and ran when Jesus was arrested in the Garden of Gethsemane (26:56), reflecting their fearful, survival-oriented denial of what was taking place.
2. Such fear-based striving for survival also was certainly the case with Peter's threefold denial (26:69–74), as mirrored in his bitter tears of realization afterward (v. 75).
3. The example of Judas Iscariot is the most profound. Though numbered among Jesus' twelve closest disciples (Matt. 10:4), Judas apparently never got beyond his denial of who Jesus really is (as seen in Matt. 26:14–16). Finally, the sense of guilt made his denial overwhelming (27:3–4)! Instead of seeking recovery, however, Judas chose to commit suicide—a tragically common outcome in extreme cases of denial.

Let's not forget, though, that there is also some highly encouraging good news. Matthew 27–28 conclusively demonstrates that *discipleship can ultimately overcome denial!*

We are introduced to Joseph of Arimathea,[19] who had been a secret disciple for some time (Matt. 27:57). In the midst of the shock of Jesus' death, he boldly "came out of the closet" and requested Jesus' body for burial in his own personal grave (vv. 58–60).

Climactically, the eleven apostles wrestled through their denial (28:16–17) before receiving the Great Commission (vv. 18–20).

How fitting for a book that has so much to say about both discipleship and denial that these, who would be the foundation of the church (Eph. 2:20), making disciples (Matt. 28:19) throughout the known world in the power of the Holy Spirit (Acts 1:8), received their final marching orders so soon after recovering from a deep bout of denial!

2

The Reality of Suffering and Recovery

Gospel of Mark

In his book *The Problem of Pain*, C. S. Lewis examines human suffering from an intellectual and philosophical perspective. In a penetrating, yet somewhat emotionally removed, manner he describes human pain succinctly and categorically. He defines the first level as "a particular kind of sensation, probably conveyed by specialised nerve fibers, and recognisable by the patient as that kind of sensation whether he dislikes it or not."[1]

The second level, Lewis states, is "any experience, whether physical or mental, which the patient dislikes."[2] It is this level that he discusses in depth throughout the rest of the book, enumerating on the various aspects of human pain and suffering.

It's not as if Lewis is misguided or unbalanced in his treatment of the problem of suffering. He speaks the truth in a brilliant and ingenious fashion. Pain, he attests, is God's way of getting our attention. Lewis communicates this fact in the following poignant statement: "But pain insists upon being attended to. God whispers to us in our pleasures, speaks in our conscience, but shouts in our pains: it is His megaphone to rouse a deaf world."[3]

It is apparent, however, as you read this profound book on the problem of pain that Lewis's approach lacks one very crucial element: personal experience. God remedied this situation by bringing Lewis into a relationship with a woman who was to undergo intense suffering. He married her, fell in love with her (yes, in that order!), and then watched her die an agonizing death.

C. S. Lewis married Joy Davidman Gresham as a mere legal formality to save her from deportation. Shortly before they were married, she was diagnosed with cancer. Miraculously, the cancer went into remission, and they began to enjoy one another's company in the deepest way. In time, they actually became emotionally what they were legally: husband and wife.

Then, tragically, at the height of their relationship, the cancer came back with a vengeance, and she died shortly thereafter. God shouted at Lewis in the pain of his devastating loss. The dreadful experience put a heart in his chest so to speak. This is evident in what he had to say about suffering after her death:

> Feelings, and feelings, and feelings. Let me try thinking instead. From the rational point of view, what new factor has H.'s death introduced into the universe? What grounds has it given me for doubting all that I believe? . . . We were even promised sufferings. They were part of the program. We were even told, "Blessed are they that mourn," and I accepted it. I've got nothing that I haven't bargained for. Of course it is different when the thing happens to oneself, not to others, and in reality, not in imagination. . . . If I had really cared, as I thought I did, about the sorrows of the world, I should not have been so overwhelmed when my own sorrow came.[4]

The Nature of Biblical Suffering

What does the life of C. S. Lewis teach us about biblical suffering? Just this: Biblical suffering is when God uses seemingly senseless human pain and ultimately transforms it into something

meaningful to accomplish his purposes for our lives and his kingdom. In other words, God is able to redeem our sufferings—when
we allow him to.

Joy Gresham, Lewis's wife, suffered intense pain in her battle
with cancer, but the disease brought her to faith in Jesus Christ.
Hence, she received the healing of her soul and eternal life. Lewis
became a shattered man through the experience, but he obtained
a faith that was deeper and richer than he ever thought possible.
God was glorified through this trial.

The fact that God can redeem human sufferings and turn
them into something meaningful is abundantly clear throughout the New Testament. The Scriptures teach us that pain and
suffering are a reality in a fallen world. When the trials of life
are submitted to the Lord or are for the Lord's sake, however,
they are not in vain. God is glorified through the sufferings and
witness of his people.

Consider the despondent woman in Mark 5:24–34. She was suffering from an ailment that no doctor could cure. In desperation
she made her way through the bustling crowd, touched the cloak
of Christ, and was instantly healed. She knew Christ had freed her
from suffering and witnessed to the crowd on his behalf (Luke 8:47).

Or how about the blind man in John 9? He was born blind so
that the work of God might be displayed in his life (9:3). The Lord
Jesus healed his eyes, and he became a testimony to his family,
to the religious leaders, and to his whole community. This man
was ultimately rejected by his loved ones (vv. 20–23, 34), but what
he received from Jesus was much more than what he lost.

Over and over again, especially throughout the Gospels, there
is a consistent theme of human suffering, healing through Christ,
and glory to God through the witness of the people. In a very real
sense, the kingdom of God was being established through the
Messiah's ministry to hurting people.

This is not to say that everyone who comes to Christ is healed
or that every wound, especially emotional, is immediately cured.
It isn't. My point is to elucidate the biblical principle that human
suffering, when submitted to the Lord, is never in vain. God's
glory should be a primary goal for the disciple of Christ, regardless of the circumstances.

Whether the suffering ends in death, as was the case with Joy Gresham, with rejection, like the blind man in John 9, or with the total acceptance experienced by the woman in Mark 5:24–34, God is working for our good and his kingdom purposes. No matter the outcome, we can never go wrong with God.

There is ultimately no escape from suffering in a fallen world. In fact, both the Lord (John 16:33) and the apostle Paul assure us that we will experience pain (Acts 14:22), but it is up to us as to how we will respond to it. We can either turn to God in faith and obedience, or we can harden our hearts against him in bitterness and anger.

For a scriptural example of these two dynamics, consider Peter and Judas. Peter denied Christ three times and suffered bitterly for what he had done (Mark 14:66–72). But he repented, and Jesus reinstated him (Mark 16:7; John 21).

Judas, on the other hand, betrayed Jesus and agonized with intense feelings of remorse. Instead of repenting and finding forgiveness, however, he ended his life (Matt. 27:3–5).

Those of us who are disciples of Christ and whose lives have been touched in the area of recovery issues can follow the example of either Peter or Judas. We can bring our sins, sufferings, and failures to God to be forgiven and redeemed. Or we can, like Judas, harden our hearts and walk the path of self-destruction. The choice is ours to make.

Whether our suffering is the direct result of our own actions or was brought on by something or someone else, Christ is willing to bear the burden with us. For no one understands human pain more than he. Therefore, he is compassionate and merciful to all who come to him in truth.

Suffering in the Lord's will finds its ultimate fulfillment at Christ's cross. His anguish and death, which seemed senseless at the time, purchased salvation for the world. In his sacrifice, he brought supreme glory to God. He is our example of suffering, submission, and obedience. As George MacDonald so aptly stated, "The Son of God suffered unto death, not that men might not suffer, but that their sufferings might be like His."[5]

This is precisely the point that Mark wanted to get across to his first century readers. They were being persecuted greatly for their faith. Because these disciples were despairing and ready to give up, Mark wrote to encourage them and to inform them that true discipleship (and recovery) is the way of the cross.

The Historical Setting of the Book of Mark

Although it is difficult to pinpoint a precise date and destination for any of the Gospels, there are a few external and internal factors that give us some clue of the life setting of the Book of Mark.

First, Irenaeus, an early church father, and early church tradition testify that Mark wrote his Gospel shortly after the martyrdom of Peter at Rome in A.D. 64.[6] It is generally held that Peter was associated with the church at Rome and that Mark received most of the information for his book from him there. This means that Mark was probably well acquainted with the Roman church, which was beginning to undergo intense persecution at that time.

As for the internal structure of Mark, suffering and persecution, especially in the life of Jesus, are prominent themes. The suffering of Jesus is evident not only in his crucifixion, but also in his ministry, his teachings, and his dealings with the disciples. It is interesting to note that Mark, who wrote the shortest Gospel, devotes one-third of it (Mark 11–16) to the last week and death of Jesus.

In light of the apparent external and internal evidence, many evangelical scholars concur that Mark was probably written to the Christians in Rome between A.D. 64 and 67. This would place the writing during the reign of Emperor Nero.[7]

Assuming that this date and destination are accurate, it sheds great light on the historical situation of the Roman Christians and on Mark's purpose for writing to them. These believers were facing desperate times, and Mark was moved to respond to their need.[8]

In A.D. 64, during Nero's reign, a terrible fire broke out in Rome, destroying almost half the city. Rumors spread that Nero himself had started the fire. In order to quell these vicious accusations, Nero fixed the blame on the Christians in Rome.

This, then, gave him a reason to greatly persecute the Roman believers. They became Nero's scapegoat so to speak. Tacitus, a first century Roman historian, describes in detail what took place at that time. I've included most of his discussion in order to show the gravity of the situation:

> But all human efforts, all the lavish gifts of the emperor, and the propitiations of the gods, did not banish the sinister belief that the conflagration was the result of an order. Consequently, to get rid of the report, Nero fastened the guilt and inflicted the most exquisite tortures on a class hated for their abominations, called Christians by the populace. . . . Accordingly, an arrest was first made of all who confessed; then, upon their information, an immense multitude was convicted, not so much of the crime of arson, as of hatred of the human race. Mockery of every sort was added to their deaths. Covered with the skins of beasts, they were torn by dogs and perished, or were nailed to crosses, or were doomed to the flames. These served to illuminate the night when daylight failed. Nero had thrown open his gardens for the spectacle, and was exhibiting a show in the circus, while he mingled with the people in the dress of a charioteer or drove about in a chariot. Hence, even for criminals who deserved extreme and exemplary punishment, there arose a feeling of compassion; for it was not, as it seemed, for the public good, but to glut one man's cruelty, that they were being destroyed.[9]

Besides giving a detailed description of the tortures endured by the Roman Christians, Tacitus gives us insight into the populace's general attitude toward them. They were known as "haters of the human race," and their practices were considered "abominable."

We must understand these accusations in their context. The Christians were mostly misunderstood by the first century pagan culture. They were considered *atheists* because they did not worship the pagan gods. They were charged with *cannibalism* because they "drank the blood and ate the flesh" of the Son of God at the Lord's Supper. They were accused of *incest* because they called themselves "brothers and sisters" and participated in "love feasts" (fellowship).[10]

Roman society misunderstood the Christians' terminology and despised them for it, but there were other reasons for the pagan culture's disdain of Christians. Chief among them was the idea of following a crucified Lord. This was a despicable concept to pagan thinking.

Persecuted and misunderstood! Does that sound familiar to those of you who are in recovery? No, you have not been falsely accused or tortured to death by the government, but you know the pain of unjust punishment. The suffering you have endured, both in the past and in the present, may seem senseless and meaningless to you.

The suffering and persecution must have seemed senseless to the Christians in the first century, too. Mark wrote his Gospel to strengthen and encourage those believers in Rome, and he speaks to suffering disciples today. It's a hard message to hear, but we must listen. Wessel sums it up beautifully in the following statement:

> [Mark] was writing a book for the guidance and support of his fellow Christians in a situation of intense crisis. . . . The way Mark prepares his Christian readers for suffering is by placing before them the passion experience of Jesus. Jesus' way was a *via dolorosa*. The way of discipleship for Christians is the same way—the way of the Cross.[11]

Jesus' Example of Suffering

Mark's Gospel teaches us many things about the life and ministry of Jesus. Yet one aspect of his personhood stands out and is made abundantly clear throughout Mark. The Son of God was not immune to suffering, and he was not distant from those who were suffering all around him.

Jesus' suffering, which found its climax at the cross, was evident throughout his ministry. Like a skilled artist, Mark paints a picture of the Son of God as the Suffering Servant. He does this primarily for two reasons:

1. to reveal Jesus' compassion and patience
2. to portray his life as an example to be followed

Jesus has paved the way of discipleship. He has gone before us so that we may follow in his footsteps, in suffering and in serving. We can take heart, however, because we do not walk this path alone. He is with us. In order to understand the suffering and serving aspects of discipleship and how they apply to recovery, let's look at a few examples from Jesus' life.

Mark gives us a vivid account of what Jesus' family thought of him and his ministry. On a particular day such a large crowd had gathered around Jesus and his disciples that they could not even eat. His family went to take charge of him because they thought he was out of his mind (Mark 3:20–21; see also vv. 31–35).

While Jesus was serving the multitude, he was suffering contempt from his family. He was misunderstood and unfairly judged by his loved ones. For us, doing the will of God may bring about the kind of treatment Jesus experienced or something even worse.

The obedience that discipleship demands may cost you the loss of respect from your earthly family. It is a high price to pay for God's kingdom, but, just like Jesus, we must count the cost and take the risk. He teaches us, by example, that there are more important things to live and die for.

Jesus assures us that we will not be alone. He offers us new relationships with fellow believers, calling them our brothers, sisters, and mothers (Mark 3:35; 10:29–31). To be sure, Jesus did not reject his earthly family, but he set higher spiritual priorities.

Christ teaches us in these verses that spiritual relationships take precedence over our earthly ones. We form his body, the church, and within this context we find the comfort of his help and presence. As Christ's body, we are eternally connected to him, and that bond should get us through times of suffering and persecution.

Woven throughout Christ's teachings concerning his impending suffering and death are references to the persecutions his followers would endure. This is no accident. Mark was communicating to his first century readers that Jesus predicted their persecutions. Therefore, they should not be surprised at suffering for their Master.

When Jesus predicted his death (Mark 8:31), he was quick to inform his disciples that anyone who would follow him must also deny himself, take up his cross, and follow him (vv. 34–36). To deny yourself in this context is to, like Jesus, put God's will before your own, no matter the consequences.

In Mark 10:32–34, Jesus once again foretold his sufferings and death. The subsequent verses give astonishing insight into the requirements of true discipleship (vv. 35–45). James and John, still not understanding the nature of Christ's ministry, made an outlandish request of him at that time. One wanted to sit at his right hand and the other at his left in his kingdom.

Jesus asked them if they were ready to endure the kind of sufferings he was about to experience. Without question, they said they were. Jesus assured them that they would indeed suffer, but they would not be guaranteed their desired position in the future. For "whoever wishes to become great among you shall be your servant; and whoever wishes to be first among you shall be slave of all" (vv. 43–44).

Jesus did not stop his discussion there. He set himself up as the example, giving them the reason behind his answer: "For even the Son of Man did not come to be served, but to serve, and to give His life a ransom for many" (v. 45).

Obedience, suffering, and serving. This was Jesus' answer to his disciples, Mark's message to his persecuted first century readers, and the same truth that reaches down through the centuries and speaks to disciples in recovery today:

1. Obedience to the will of God should be first and foremost in the life of a disciple.
2. Suffering will come to followers of Christ and should be expected.
3. Serving the Lord and others should be an integral part of a disciple's life, regardless of the consequences.

Suffering for the Lord's sake, whether the pain is emotional, physical, or spiritual, is never in vain. Those who are obedient will ultimately "receive a hundred times as much now in the present age, houses and brothers and sisters and mothers and children and farms, *along with persecutions;* and in the age to come, eternal life" (Mark 10:30, italics mine).

These statements offer great encouragement to those who are being purified in the recovery process. We can also take heart in knowing that if we have not yet achieved the radical commitment commanded by Christ for discipleship, he is patient with our failings. He demonstrated that clearly through his dealings with his disciples.

The Disciples' Failure and Recovery

Jesus' first disciples were anything but perfectly successful in following their Lord. Their failure and their recovery are both needed examples in understanding how recovery dovetails with discipleship. There are at least two aspects of the disciples' lives that display their failures and reveal Christ's patience in dealing with them.

Failure to Comprehend the Nature of Christ's Mission

It's easy to understand why the disciples were so obtuse about the purpose of their Lord's mission. After all, there had never been anyone quite like Jesus! Still, Peter and the gang had been given plenty of opportunities to learn something about his person. Was it a lack of faith in him or a lack of insight about their own nature that caused their dullness? As it turns out, it was a little of both.

Take, for example, the incident that took place on the Sea of Galilee in Mark 4:35–41. Jesus and the disciples were crossing over to the other side of the sea when a furious storm suddenly came upon them. The disciples, gripped with fear, woke Jesus up and said, "Teacher, do You not care that we are perishing?" (v. 38).

In a moment of trial, they questioned the character of their Lord. By this time the disciples had on many occasions witnessed Christ's power, love, and compassion for troubled people (see Mark 1:23–25, 32–34; 2:1–12; 3:1–6, 10–11). Surely they must have known their Lord cared about them (and himself!) in their time of trouble.

The Lord Jesus, with a word, quieted the storm and rebuked his disciples for their lack of faith. Their doubt caused them to question the integrity of Jesus. Afterward, they were even more baffled about his identity. Their confusion about him and his ministry continued to grow as they walked with him through the dusty streets of Judea.

Consider the lively conversation the disciples witnessed between Jesus and the Pharisees in Mark 7:1–23. The disciples were being criticized by the Pharisees for failing to ceremonially cleanse their hands before eating. Jesus quickly pointed out the Pharisees' hypocrisy and, in the process, exposed the wickedness residing in every human heart (vv. 6–7, 14–15).

Jesus explained to the crowd that what makes human beings unclean is the sinful heart, not unclean hands. Evil is primarily due to inside factors, not outside forces. Still the disciples did not understand this concept. When Jesus entered the house, they asked him about it.

He answered them by beginning with a question: "Are you so lacking in understanding also?" (v. 18). Then he proceeded to list the various sins that flow from the heart and defile the man (vv. 20–23). The disciples, unaware of the condition of their own hearts, misunderstood Jesus' teaching.

On this occasion it was not a lack of faith in Jesus that caused the problem but a lack of insight concerning their own nature. We can clearly see both of these dynamics at work in the lives of the disciples throughout the Book of Mark.[12]

Failure to Support Christ in His Hour of Need

It was Christ's last Passover meal. He and his closest disciples were celebrating it with joy in that large upper room (Mark 14:12–31), and they, as always, felt safe and secure in his presence. It was easy for them to be brave under such circumstances.

Even when Jesus revealed to the disciples that they would all fall away from him and that Peter would deny him three times, the disciples insisted on their steadfast commitment to him. "Peter kept saying insistently, 'Even if I have to die with You, I will not deny You!' And they all were saying the same thing, too" (Mark 14:31).

Then they came to the Garden of Gethsemane (14:32–41). That place had an uncanny ability to test the heart, its vows and convictions. Jesus desperately needed his friends to walk through that Gethsemane experience with him, but he suffered, agonized, and persevered alone.

The disciples fell asleep. Jesus came and woke them once, but their eyes were too heavy, and they just couldn't stay awake (vv. 37–41). Then Judas came with an angry crowd carrying swords and clubs. When they bound Jesus to take him away, his weary disciples gathered their strength, "left Him and fled" (v. 50).

Finally, Peter, following Jesus at a distance, entered the courtyard of the high priest. There he three times denied he knew Christ. When Peter realized what he had done, he was overwhelmed with grief, went outside, and wept bitterly (14:54, 66–72).

So, as you can see, we are not alone in our constant battle with failure. The Book of Mark is full of examples of the failures of those who were closest to Christ—his disciples. In many ways, twentieth century disciples in the recovery process (every disciple of Christ, to some extent), struggle with the same failures the first disciples did.

Think about it. Have you ever questioned the character of your Lord in the moment of trial? Have you accused him falsely because it seemed as though he was sleeping through your hour of need? Have you felt his gentle rebuke for your lack of faith and understanding? Worse yet, have you ever betrayed him, deserted him, or denied him?

We all have, at one time or another, been guilty of such things. The good news is that Jesus is the God of the second chance. He heals, restores, and strengthens his faltering disciples.

In Mark 16:7, the angel told the women who were mourning at Jesus' tomb to go and "tell His disciples and Peter, 'He is going before you into Galilee; there you will see Him, just as He said to you.'" Jesus singled out Peter, the one who was closest to him and the one who probably hurt him the most, and reinstated him. He let those women know that Peter was still one of his.

Max Lucado summed up this situation beautifully when he wrote, "It's not every day that you find someone who will give you a second chance—much less someone who will give you a second chance every day. But in Jesus, Peter found both."[13]

We too can experience the same grace Peter and the disciples did. In the beginning, those disciples fell short of the radical commitment to discipleship the Lord commanded. But as the Book of Acts and early church tradition bears out, they all became what the Lord intended them to be: radically committed disciples.

What was their secret? The power of Christ flowed through their lives, in sufferings and persecutions. They learned the value of suffering for his sake. They no longer ran from the pain of being associated with his name.

The Value of Biblical Suffering

The New Testament writers speak much about suffering. It is seen by them not as something to be avoided but as something to be expected as a natural part of living the Christian life (e.g., Rom. 5:3; Phil. 1:29; 2 Thess. 1:5; James 1:2–3; 1 Peter 4:12–13). They learned from experience the intrinsic value of suffering for Jesus' sake.

From a personal viewpoint, there are at least four reasons why we should embrace our present sufferings.

Suffering Shatters Self-Sufficiency

For me, the crumbling of my self-reliance seemed like no benefit at all. I liked to be in control. I took pride in my rugged independence. However, the value I placed on my self-sufficient lifestyle blinded me to the fact that I was standing on shifting sand.

I had to learn a valuable lesson the hard way. During the writing of this chapter, I lost a child to miscarriage in my third month of pregnancy. When I went to the doctor on a routine prenatal visit, he found no heartbeat and later informed me that the baby was dead.

Through the searching questions and what seemed like endless grief, I came to the end of myself. I no longer valued my so-called strength and self-sufficiency. It was the one good thing that came out of this tragedy. It shattered my "ideal" self-image.

Suffering Unmasks Our Pretenses

Suffering brings about self-examination in the deepest sense. It stripped away all the fluff in my life and laid bare the naked truth of who I really was. The many disguises I used to hide my weaknesses suddenly melted away in the heat of this fiery trial.

My miscarriage caused me to reevaluate myself and my priorities. I wanted to be who I really was and live for what really mattered. Being honest with myself and my weaknesses revolutionized and revitalized my relationship with the Lord. The pain drove me to the throne of grace, which was the best possible place I could go.

Suffering Brings Us to God

I knew intellectually that death is an integral part of living in a fallen world, but, much like C. S. Lewis, I never knew death experientially. It was the most difficult thing I've ever lived through, but the experience profoundly impacted me and changed me—for the good.

Yes, the personal pain and suffering associated with losing a baby could have potentially hardened me to God. I realize that I may still go through stages of anger, disillusionment, and grief in which I distance myself from him for a while.

Nevertheless, I am confident that my deep need for God's comfort and the soothing love of his Holy Spirit will draw me to him again and again. I have discovered that suffering has an ironic and mysterious way of revealing our greatest weaknesses and yet producing in us true spiritual strength. In other words, biblical suffering produces holy character.

Suffering Causes True Spiritual Growth

Suffering purifies and refines the soul. My recent loss has taught me something of the cost of true discipleship and recovery. The paths, often bordered by sorrow and suffering, wind through many hills and valleys. They gently and sometimes forcefully lead us directly to the cross of Christ. He is our model and our true source of temporal, and ultimately eternal, recovery.

The Book of Mark clearly shows us that we are on our way to spiritual maturity when we can honestly grasp the hands of sorrow and suffering and let them teach us the way of discipleship. Through my own suffering and loss, I am slowly learning to do just that.

3

Calling All Outcasts and Sinners!

Gospel of Luke

It had been one of those tiresome and uneventful nights—the kind that seemed to last forever. The weary fishermen could not understand it. They used the same procedure this night as they did every other night. They rowed out to deep waters, let down their dragnet, and waited. On this particular night, however, their patience and hard efforts were met with still waters and empty nets. They couldn't wait for sunrise and time to quit.

The Dawning of Day and Insight

As the early sunlight finally began to illuminate the eastern sky, the dispirited fishermen hastily made their way toward shore. Much to their surprise, the seaside, usually vacant in the early morning, was filled with people. They were all crowding around Jesus, that popular Galilean preacher.

Jesus, being smothered by this crowd, immediately stepped into Simon Peter's boat, put out from shore, and taught the people the Word of God. When he finished, he quickly dismissed the multitude, turned to Peter, and said, "Put out into the deep water and let down your nets for a catch" (Luke 5:4). Peter must have looked shocked and bewildered. He must have thought, "What does this rabbi know about fishing?"

Nevertheless, he reverently responded to Jesus' request: "Master, we worked hard all night and caught nothing, but at Your bidding I will let down the nets" (Luke 5:5). Then Peter's jaw dropped! What a catch! His boat could hardly hold the nets full of fish. It seemed that the Preacher might really know a thing or two about fishing. Or could it also have been that the fish themselves knew something about the one who summoned them? Something that Peter himself was about to learn?

This enormous catch of fish evoked a peculiar response from this soon-to-be disciple: "Depart from me, for I am a sinful man, O Lord!" (v. 8). The voice of Jesus, a boat full of fish, and Peter somehow realized his sinfulness. The voice of Jesus drew fish from deep waters, and it also brought to light the dark side of Peter's heart. This is the exact response Jesus was waiting for. Now Peter was ready for the call.

Jesus said to him, "Do not fear, from now on you will be catching men" (v. 10). Peter's heart had been exposed, and now his future vocation was revealed. The catch of fish was an incredible witness to Christ's power and authority. Like the fish, Peter was literally drawn to his call. He left everything and followed Jesus (v. 11).

In time, Peter was to discover just how much this Galilean Preacher knew about fishing. His first lesson was his own experience. He, a simple fisherman, was caught by Jesus, the true Fisher of men. Peter was to continue to learn, by Jesus' enduring example, the incredible scriptural art of catching men.

Calling Society's Scuzballs

Peter's second teachable moment came shortly after he docked his boat and hung up his nets. Jesus was walking along one day when he spotted Matthew, a tax collector, sitting at his booth.

Jesus said to him, "Follow me." And Matthew, like Peter, left everything and followed him (Luke 5:27–28).

Jesus' call to Matthew must have really surprised Peter. Fishermen may not have been highly esteemed in society, but at least
they were accepted. Tax collectors, on the other hand, were an
accursed brood! Often accused of being collaborators with the
Roman government, they were not well liked by their fellow Jews.
The Pharisees and the teachers of law especially disdained them
and considered them religious outcasts.

Immediately after Matthew's call to discipleship, he welcomed
Jesus into his home and held a great banquet in his honor (Luke
5:29). Matthew invited his fellow tax collectors to join them in
the celebration. In the first century Jewish culture, table fellowship indicated intimate relations and mutual identification.[1] Eating together strongly signified a closeness and a bond between
the participants.

This unnerved the Pharisees, and they severely criticized Jesus
for eating "with the tax-gatherers and sinners" (v. 30). Notice that
in Luke's account Jesus did not deny their sinfulness nor the fact
that they could have been considered religious outcasts. Instead
he said, "I have not come to call the righteous but sinners to repentance" (Luke 5:32).

Peter, a self-proclaimed sinful fisherman, and Matthew, a tax
collector, a religious outcast, and an accused sinner, found purpose and acceptance from the one who came to call them to repentance. Jesus' call to repentance evidently did not threaten them.
It is interesting to note that Luke records no negative reaction
from the disciples to Jesus' "repentance" statement.

In fact, Peter and Matthew seemed eager to change their mind
(repent) and embark on the road to discipleship. Unfortunately,
today the word *repentance* often carries with it negative connota-
tions. This is justifiable to some extent because, in certain evangelical circles, the word has often been used as a weapon rather
than an invitation.

As a result, outcasts and sinners of today often take offense at
Jesus' message of repentance. They feel judged or condemned by
it. They are not eager to leave everything and follow him. Many
modern-day would-be disciples, especially those in the process of

recovery, do not feel worthy of such a calling—the high calling of repentance and discipleship.

Nevertheless, it remains true that repentance is a necessary prerequisite to discipleship and recovery. Both require a change of mind and heart. The calling of Peter and Matthew in Luke 5:1–32 indicates that repentance should be understood as a good thing. It brings us into intimate fellowship with God and others and ushers us into a brand-new way of life. It is the doorway to the kingdom of God.

Maybe you feel like Peter first did at his calling, ever so aware of your sinfulness in the presence of Jesus. Covered in your shame, you also have told the Lord to depart from you (Mark 5:8). Or perhaps you can identify with Matthew, who was considered a social and religious outcast, unknown and unacceptable to just about everyone.

You have plenty of reason for hope today if you feel like a Peter or a Matthew. Jesus came for people like you (and me), for sinners and outcasts. He came "to seek and to save that which was lost" (Luke 19:10). This includes twentieth century believers, who are just as helpless as those in the first century.

The good news is that just as Jesus called Peter, Matthew, and the other disciples to repent and follow him, so he is calling us today. The invitation to repent and become a disciple goes out to all people in every generation: to the Jew and Gentile, to the slave and free, to the high class and the low class, and to people who struggle with all kinds of emotional issues.

No one is forgotten or excluded! The one who is willing to count the cost, accept the message, and follow Christ will never be turned away. This is the message Luke wanted to communicate to his first century readers. It is equally a message of hope and encouragement to disciples today who wrestle with feelings of insecurity and unworthiness.

The Setting of the Book of Luke

Luke is the only Gospel that is actually addressed to an individual—to the "most excellent Theophilus" (Luke 1:3). This title, "most excellent," indicates that Theophilus was probably a member of the upper class in Roman society, possibly a government official. He may have even sponsored the writing project—a common practice in first century Roman culture.[2]

Apparently, Theophilus had some doubts or at least a few questions concerning what he had been taught about the Christian faith. Luke was writing so that this honorable man "might know the exact truth about the things [he had] been taught" (Luke 1:4). Theophilus's concerns were understandable in view of the many rival religions that existed during that period of the Roman Empire.

Luke's address to Theophilus in the prologue, along with his sophisticated literary style, has led many scholars to believe that he was writing primarily to high-class, well-educated Greek or Greek-speaking believers.[3] It's possible that these Christians may not have been completely informed about their faith and had a desire to know more about its exact origins. If this explanation is accurate, it gives us some idea of Luke's overall purpose for writing.

To give assurance to Theophilus (and, by implication, to others) concerning the reliability of the Christian faith was certainly one of Luke's purposes for writing. But it should probably be viewed as his narrow purpose. Because Luke covers such a wide range of topics in his Gospel, it would be inadequate to limit his overall goal to the apparent inquiries of Theophilus and others.

There is a much broader goal evident throughout Luke's Gospel, which culminates in his second volume, the Book of Acts.[4] That is the *universality of salvation*. His pressing message is that the gospel transcends all racial and socioeconomic barriers. It is good news for all people in every generation.

While both the narrow and broad purposes of the Book of Luke are vitally important to our faith, it is the latter that holds special significance and encouragement for disciples in recovery. Luke's focus on the universality of salvation is our hope of unconditional love and acceptance. This wider purpose assures us of God's concern for *all* people, regardless of their condition.

Luke stresses the universality of salvation in a variety of ways throughout his Gospel. Leon Morris, in his commentary on Luke, shows just how prevalent this theme is:

Luke tells us that the message of the angel concerned people in general, not specially Israel (2:14). He takes the genealogy of Jesus right back to Adam (3:38), the progenitor of mankind. . . . He tells us about Samaritans, for example when the disciples wanted to call down fire on them (9:51–54), or in the parable of the Good Samaritan (10:30–37), or in the information that the grateful leper was of this race (17:16). He refers to Gentiles in the song of Simeon (2:32) and tells us that Jesus spoke approvingly of non-Israelites such as the widow of Zarephath and Naaman the Syrian (4:25–27). He tells us about the healing of a centurion's slave (7:2–10). He records words about people coming from all the directions of the compass to sit in God's kingdom (13:29) and the great commission that the gospel be preached to all nations (24:47) . . . It is clear that Luke has a deep interest in God's concern for all people.[5]

Morris reveals two important things about Luke's approach to the subject of universal salvation. First, the topic of salvation functions as literary bookends in Luke's Gospel. From the angel's announcement of the Savior's birth in 2:10 to the Savior's description of the Great Commission in 24:47, Luke begins and ends his book with the idea of universal salvation.

Second, Luke introduces people from undesirable and poor social backgrounds to emphasize the impartiality of the salvation message. Gentiles, Samaritans, widows, slaves, and lepers fill the pages of Luke's Gospel. The impartiality and universality of salvation are the two most obvious themes throughout his book.

Luke consistently emphasizes Jesus' compassion toward those who populated the most despised and forgotten elements of society. His focus on the downtrodden is extraordinary, especially in light of the fact that his original audience may have been primarily of the upper class. Could it be that Luke was subtly exhorting them to show true compassion toward *all* people, rich or poor, even as their Lord did?

Jesus and the Recovery of the Sinful Forgotten

Jesus Christ, the Son of God, had a clearly defined mission to accomplish. He came:

to preach the gospel to the poor . . . to proclaim release to the cap-
tives, and recovery of sight to the blind, to set free those who are
downtrodden, to proclaim the favorable year of the Lord. . . . to
seek and to save that which was lost.

Luke 4:18–19; 19:10

Jesus came not as a condemning judge or conquering hero,
however, but as a helpless, vulnerable babe in a manger.[6] His birth
drew no unusual attention. If it weren't for the animals and a few
shepherds, the day would have passed by virtually unnoticed. It
was a day destined to be forgotten.

The amazing irony is that this obscure birth of a peasant's child
changed the course of human history! What is even more absurd
is the significance of his birthplace. As Frederick Buechner so
poignantly described it, Jesus' inconspicuous birthplace represents
God's relentless pursuit of humankind in a most striking way:

Those who believe in God can never in a way be sure of him again.
Once they have seen him in a stable, they can never be sure where
he will appear or to what lengths he will go or to what ludicrous
depths of self-humiliation he will descend in his wild pursuit of man.
If holiness and the awful power and majesty of God are present in
this least auspicious of all events, this birth of a peasant's child, then
there is no place or time so lowly and earthbound but that holiness
can be present there too. And this means that we are never safe, that
there is no place where we can hide from God, no place where we
are safe from his power to break in two and recreate the human heart
because it is just where he seems most helpless that he is most strong,
and just where we least expect him that he comes most fully.

For those who believe in God, it means, this birth, that God himself is never safe from us, and maybe that is the dark side of Christ-
mas, the terror of the silence. He comes in such a way that we can
always turn him down, as we could crack the baby's skull like an
eggshell or nail him up when he gets too big for that. . . . The child
is born in the night—the mother's exhausted flesh, the father's face
clenched like a fist—and nothing is ever the same again.[7]

Christ's unpresuming birth and inauspicious birthplace reveal
in a remarkable way God's love and concern for the forgotten. He

will descend to the deepest, darkest places of the earth to recover lost humanity. In essence, Christ's humble beginnings prepared him for his earthly ministry to the forgotten. He was able to completely empathize with the lonely, the brokenhearted, and the despised outcast.

Jesus himself was "despised and forsaken of men, a man of sorrows, and acquainted with grief" (Isa. 53:3). He put himself at our mercy, making himself vulnerable to our cruelty, not only in his birth but throughout his ministry and death, in order to fully enter into the human experience. He identified with suffering humanity on every level.[8]

It is no surprise, then, that the hurting and afflicted people of Jesus' day were drawn to him. He sought them out, and they responded to his voice like sheep without a shepherd. And that is precisely what many of them were. Aimlessly, they wandered on the hills of Judea, wallowing in the muck and mire of their lives until he called them. And, like a Good Shepherd, Jesus gathered them up and cared for them. He recovered his lost sheep (Luke 15:3–7).

Luke's Gospel gives many examples of the Savior rescuing and caring for hurting people. Luke does this not to make his future readers jealous but to demonstrate that God, through the person of his Son, is in touch with the needs of *all* humanity. This recovering ministry of Christ did not end in the first century.

Jesus called his first disciples in Luke 5:1–31. He steadfastly taught them the principles of discipleship, as Luke's entire Gospel bears out. Then in Luke 24:45–49, he commissioned them to carry on his work. The Book of Acts testifies that the disciples did indeed continue in Christ's work, and disciples today still carry on his ministry through the church, which is empowered by the Holy Spirit.[9]

Luke's obvious emphasis on Christ's ministry to sinners and outcasts strengthens his overall argument on the universality and impartiality of salvation. The people described in Luke's Gospel are in many ways like you and me—they loved, they laughed, they cried, and they hurt. Luke intends for us to vividly see ourselves mirrored in their lives. We can then learn from their interaction with Jesus some valuable lessons about discipleship and recovery.

Consider the sinful woman who approached Jesus at the Pharisee's house (Luke 7:36–50). She was probably a prostitute or at least a woman known to be morally loose. Jesus was reclining at the table when she came to him and anointed his feet with expensive perfume and her own tears. The Pharisees were disgusted by this act and criticized both Jesus and the woman.

This woman was obviously a sinner, the Pharisees retorted, and this man, who was supposed to be a prophet, seemed to have no clue about her moral state (v. 39)! But Jesus knew a great deal about the sinful condition of her heart. He had freely forgiven her many sins, and she accepted it. The love she lavished on him was proof of this.

The Pharisees' own wretched souls were not hidden from Christ either. He pointed out in the parable of the two debtors that their lack of love showed their hard-heartedness and insensitivity (vv. 41–47).

Consider also Zaccheus, the chief tax collector introduced to us in Luke 19:1–10. Like Matthew, Zaccheus was greatly disliked by his people. His position as chief tax collector afforded him wealth, which undoubtedly gave the people a double reason to abhor him.

One day Zaccheus heard that Jesus was about to pass through Jericho. He wanted to see him but could not, because he was short and the crowd was blocking his view. So he ran ahead of everyone, climbed a sycamore tree, and eagerly waited for Jesus to pass by (vv. 1–4).

When Jesus came to the tree, he looked up and said, "Zaccheus, hurry and come down, for today I must stay at your house" (v. 5). It's almost as if Jesus was watching for him in that tree. It's as if he purposed to go through Jericho just to stay at the house of this notorious sinner. The self-righteous Jews accompanying Jesus quickly condemned him for being "the guest of a man who is a sinner" (v. 7).

That day Zaccheus gladly opened his house and his heart to his honored guest. He did not weep over Jesus as the sinful woman did, but his words were just as moving. Zaccheus openly confessed his wrongdoing to Jesus, and the Lord responded with acceptance and forgiveness. Salvation had come to this man. The lost sinner had been found by the seeking Savior (vv. 9–10).

These two scenes communicate two very important principles relevant to discipleship and recovery:

1. *Repentance is a foundational part of the discipleship and recovery process.* At some level, both the sinful woman and Zaccheus must have examined their lives and realized their sin and need. Therefore, they had a change of heart (repented) and came to the one who could set them straight and satisfy their emptiness.

2. *Self-righteous, critical people may attempt to intimidate and hinder our pursuit of Christ, the one who calls us into discipleship and recovery.* The self-righteous Jews and Pharisees, with their snide remarks and condemning accusations, tried to keep the sinful woman and Zaccheus away from Christ—but they could not. Jesus' ministry to hurting people proved to these two sinners that he came for them and that he would not turn them away. They knew they were free to approach him openly and honestly.

True repentance is a necessary prerequisite for both discipleship and recovery. It is a required element for holy transformation to begin. God always rewards true repentance with complete forgiveness and total acceptance. Don't let the self-righteous Pharisees in your life keep you from the forgiveness and recovery offered to you in Christ!

By all means, if you, like the sinful woman, have to come uninvited to a banquet in order to communicate with Christ, then do it. Or if you have to climb a tree like Zaccheus did in order to see him, then do it. Remember, Jesus is always watching and waiting for you too.

Jesus is in the business of recovering and recruiting the lost, but his high call to discipleship is not without cost. Luke warns us that lifelong discipleship will demand nothing less than everything we have (Luke 14:16–35). This is very similar to decisions that must be made in the recovery process. While Luke compassionately depicts the inclusion of outcasts and sinners into God's plan of salvation, he also skillfully warns us of the high cost of Christ's call—something we must keep in mind as we travel on the road to biblical recovery.

Those who are in the recovery process must count the cost of facing the painful truth about themselves, even as all of Christ's disciples must deal with the consequences of walking with him who is the Truth. Needless to say, this discipleship and recovery process can be a difficult and painful experience at times. We can often feel discouraged on the journey.

Long ago Jesus' hands built and crafted the wood in his father's carpentry shop. Today those same hands are fashioning us, and this Carpenter's ultimate goal is to shape truth and holiness in our inmost being.

I wrote "The Carpenter" several years ago. As you read it, may it encourage you to know that the Master's hand is always on you, for good and not for evil. When we suffer through tremendous trials, we begin to feel as though God has lost touch with us. His workings in our lives don't always make sense. Yet the merciful, unseen Architect is in complete control, mysteriously using our pain to rebuild and shape our shattered lives.

We must not forget Luke's recorded words of Jesus:

> The Spirit of the Lord is upon Me,
> Because He anointed Me to preach the gospel to the poor.
> He has sent Me to proclaim release to the captives,
> And recovery of sight to the blind,
> To set free those who are downtrodden,
> To proclaim the favorable year of the Lord.
>
> Luke 4:18–19

So walk on in his strength, trusting in his perpetual ministry to you, the hurting!

The Carpenter

Yes, I too used to feel rejected, worthless, and unloved until I met a man who changed my life. I found out that he had been trying to introduce himself to me for quite a while, but I never had the time. One day, however, I happened to be in a place where there were some people who knew him very well. They introduced me to him.

He was different from anyone else I'd ever met. He had a deep love and compassion in his eyes, and he seemed to genuinely care about me. He was a carpenter by trade, and I noticed something very different about the way in which he did his work.

While all the other carpenters were using the finest, brand-new wood to build with, he would go to the old wood pile in the backyard and pick the most broken, marred, and abused wood he could find. He would take that old abused wood and build the most beautiful statues with it. Indeed, their beauty surpassed that of any of the other carpenters' work.

I ask him why he took the marred, abused wood to work with instead of the new. He smiled at me warmly, and with a sparkle in his eye he said, "love to take the marred, the abused,wood he could find. He would take that old abused wood and build the most beautiful statues with it. Indeed, their beauty surpassed that of any of the other carpenters' work.

I asked him why he took the marred, abused wood to work with instead of the new. He smiled at me warmly, and with a sparkle in his eye he said, "love to take the marred, the abused, the unwanted, the rejected and make something beautiful. . . . That is what I do best."

Somehow i sensed he was talking about more than just wood. The more time I spent with him, the more I realized how true this feeling was. You see, he taught me so much about myself. Indeed, he knew me much better than I knew myself. It's as if I stood transparent before him, but I felt no shame.

His compassion and love seemed to have no end, He reached out to anyone and everyone who was around him. He had many friends, and I noticed something very familiar about the friends he chose. They were much like the wood he chose to work with: abused, marred, rejected, and unwanted. They were the lonely and discarded of society.

He loved his special friends so much, and they loved him. There was a glorious light that shone in their faces just from being in his presence. Because of him, they now had each other. And I am not ashamed to say that I am one of them.

I have never felt so loved and accepted.

One day, though, out of desperate curiosity, I had to ask him, "Sir, why do you care so much? How could you love us when no one else does?"

He looked at me with the compassion that was now so familiar and said, "Friend, I too was abused, marred, rejected, and unwanted. I know what it's like. They hung me on a marred, broken piece of wood on a lonely mountainside two thousand years ago.

"But I have come back from the dead to build my church out of the broken, the abused, and the rejected. I will make them into a people for myself. As the marred wood in my hands becomes beautiful and useful, so will my people be."

This Carpenter from Galilee gave me the greatest most precious gift of all—himself.

His name is Jesus.

4

That You May Believe . . .

Gospel of John

The sun was setting. A cool, evening breeze was beginning to blow through Priscilla's flower-filled garden. It was the end of another ordinary day, and she was in the kitchen preparing supper. She had removed the fish from her stone oven and was busy putting the finishing touches on her favorite vegetable dish.

The rear court was filled with the aroma of her freshly baked bread. The smell was beginning to make her hungry. The table in the garden patio was beautifully set with Priscilla's best earthenware. It was just waiting to be occupied by herself, her husband, and their three children.

"Where are those children of mine?" Priscilla thought as she watched the steam fade from the baked fish and vegetable dish she had just prepared. She walked into the central court and called out their names, "Julia, Rufus, Apelles! Dinner is ready and it's getting cold!"

"We're coming, Mom!" her oldest daughter, Julia, shouted back. "Can Mary and Hermes stay for dinner?"

Priscilla, much to her daughter's surprise, answered her question quickly, "Yes, they can stay. Hurry up now, it's getting colder by the minute!" Priscilla knew from past experience that her teenage daughter would make this request. Only this time she was not going to be caught off guard. She had gladly fixed enough food for everybody.

"Pass the bread, please," said Apelles, the youngest of Priscilla's three children. Then he stretched out his tiny arm to receive the basket. He was reclining at the far end of the table near the place his father usually reclined. Noticing that it was rapidly getting dark and his father had not yet come home, Apelles asked his mother, "Where's Dad?"

"He had to work late tonight, Honey," she responded.

"Again?" sighed Apelles. Priscilla tried hard not to notice the disappointment in her young son's eyes.

Quickly changing the subject, Priscilla asked her daughter's dinner guest a question: "How are your parents, Mary?"

"They're doing alright, I guess," she timidly replied. "I don't see them that much. Dad works a lot, and Mom spends most of her time out in the field. There's been a lot going on in our family lately and . . . well, everyone is keeping busy." Priscilla sipped her wine and listened with concern as Mary offered more information than her simple inquiry warranted.

"My older sister's husband is getting a divorce and leaving her and their two children. My brother has left home, and we don't know where he is. Mom is upset, and Dad won't talk about it."

"I'm sorry to hear that, Mary," Priscilla said, her voice revealing the sadness and confusion she was feeling.

In an attempt to bring some hope into this despairing conversation, Julia began to speak about the trials and victories that took place in the family who lived next door to them. "Our neighbors were going through a hard time too. The father worked long hours as a slave laborer. He barely made enough money to provide for the family. The mother was very sick and unable to take care of the home. This was hard on the family. They fought all the time— about money, about household duties, about life.

"Then their daughter Eunice was raped by one of the soldiers. It was terrible. She's doing okay now. But, surprisingly, this tragedy pulled the family together. They hardly fight anymore. They still have money problems. The mom still gets sick a lot. But they're sticking together. Don't worry, Mary. Things will get better for your family too."

"I'm sure it will," Mary confidently replied. But her doubtful heart was revealed by the look on her face. A disturbing silence fell upon everyone who was reclining at the table. Priscilla was astonished by the words that flowed from Julia's mouth. Her teenage daughter was obviously touched by what had happened in that neighboring family. She was not even aware that Julia was concerned about such things.

"I didn't know she was so sensitive," Priscilla thought to herself as she stared off into the distance. "But, of course, I've been so preoccupied with . . . I wonder if it bothers her when Paul and I . . ."

"Mom, can I go to the gladiator combats with Hermes tonight?" Rufus, her middle son blurted out, breaking the silence.

Priscilla was startled out of her deep thought. "You're interrupting us, Rufus! Julia, Mary, and I were talking."

"It didn't look like that to me!" Rufus snapped back. "It looked like you were sleeping with your eyes open! What were you . . ."

Priscilla abruptly broke in, cutting her son off in midsentence, "You know I don't approve of what goes on in that amphitheater."

"Come on, Mom! I'll close my eyes during the gory parts!" Rufus and Hermes were anxious to go, but Priscilla was hesitant to give her son permission to view such so-called "entertainment." On the other hand, she did not want to embarrass him in front of his friend.

"Mom, the soldiers do worse things to people out on the streets! At least the gladiators enter these games by their own choice! They know what they're in for!" Rufus retorted in one final attempt to persuade his mother. Finally, she consented and let him go.

Priscilla knew that her son's statement about the soldiers' cruel conduct was painfully true. But this did not condone the gladiators' grotesque practices. All told, she did not like what was happening in her world. Society was becoming increasingly chaotic and corrupt. Sex and violence was highly esteemed in her culture.

The gods weren't helping matters either. In fact, they were often the catalyst for further demoralization!

The Greek and Roman philosophies were devoid of hope. All of the belief systems seemed powerless to stop the evils pervading the metropolis. Her faith in the local deities left her empty and forlorn. She felt they had betrayed her trust time and again. She wondered if there was anything worth believing in.

The environment Priscilla lived in was insecure, unstable, and morally perverse. The government was crooked and uncaring. Poor economic conditions were afflicting the common people. Adultery was becoming a culturally accepted practice. As a result of the widespread turmoil, immorality and licentiousness were taking a toll on family relationships, and broken homes were quickly becoming commonplace.

Where was Priscilla to turn? Everything she had trusted in was now failing her. She wanted answers. She desperately needed hope. She was searching for something to believe in, but to no avail. The people she loved and the things she cared about were being overwhelmed by darkness. She wondered if life could ever be different. Was there anything or anybody who could truly change things?

The Purpose of John's Gospel

The apostle John's answer to Priscilla's searching questions was a resounding *yes!* The basis for this hope is found in his statement, "And the Word became flesh, and dwelt among us, and we beheld His glory, glory as of the only begotten from the Father, full of grace and truth" (John 1:14). In the midst of a dark and chaotic world, this living Word, clothed in human flesh, came to shed light on the human heart and give hope to the hopeless. This is the message of John's Gospel.

While the preceding story is purely fictional, it is a fair representation of what daily life was like among the Gentiles in the first century.[1] The problems they faced and the trials they endured were similar to ours in many ways. There is plenty of reason to believe that these first century folks suffered the same kind of physical and emotional losses we often do, for they struggled with the same complexities of life.

Bad economic conditions, poor governmental leadership, crime, divorce, and family strife are just some of the commonalities. Further study of first century metropolitan life would likely uncover many more parallels. These suffice, though, to show that life is fragile and difficult, whether it is the first century or the twentieth. Life's hardships transcend the boundaries of time, plaguing every society to a greater or lesser degree in every age.

While there were certainly some classic examples of goodness, love, and honesty sprinkled throughout Greco-Roman society, Dana concludes his investigation into the public world of the first century with this sobering statement: "In the light of all the evidence we can but conclude that society of the first century was frightfully corrupt. Indulgence was taken for granted, license was condoned, and greed was the accepted rule of life."[2]

His overall research into the private affairs of Greco-Roman life presented him with an equally dismal situation: "The birth-rate decreased, marriage became infrequent, and the home became the instrument or occasion of lust. Divorce was undoubtedly very prevalent, for, among the papyrus remains, one of the most abundant classes of documents is the divorce certificates."[3]

This was the world that John wanted to reach through his Gospel. Many of the people of that time were like Priscilla—hurting, broken, and searching for answers. The apostle John proclaimed to these first century people the glorious truth concerning God's Son. It gave them hope. His timeless message reaches down through the ages and extends the same hope to us.

The apostle John gives his readers in every generation a unique, eternal perspective on the Christ event. Unlike Matthew and Luke, John does not begin with the manger but with eternity, with the Word becoming flesh (John 1:14). Hence, his Gospel surpasses the Synoptics[4] in depth of theological insight and further elucidates the distinct nature of God's beloved Son.

John focuses on Christ's deity but does not neglect his humanity. The divine majesty of Christ is clearly displayed in John's Gospel by seven great signs (see John 2:1–12; 4:46–54; 5:1–14; 6:1–15, 19–24; 9:1–34; 11:1–46). To be sure, the apostle's overall portrayal of Christ is high and lofty, but he does not present him as unapproachable or aloof. Jesus was not out of touch with the real world in which he lived. In fact, he came so that this world might believe in him.

This is the purpose for which John wrote his Gospel: "But these have been written that you may believe that Jesus is the Christ, the Son of God; and that believing you may have life in His name" (20:31).[5] Unquestionably, belief is one of the most prominent themes woven throughout the fabric of John's book. Every other theme disclosed seems to support this dominant theme of belief.

With striking evidence of Christ's divine authority, John compels his readers to believe and obey the one who came to redeem them. The hungry hearts of the first century were ready for such a life-changing message. People like Priscilla were primed and waiting for some good news to rekindle their hope. They were to find it in John's Gospel.

It is important to understand the context into which the gospel of Jesus Christ first came. It helps us to understand our own need. When we fully realize that we are no different from the first recipients of this message, that we too are susceptible to temptations and beset with weaknesses, then we will realize our own need to believe and trust Jesus Christ. Belief and trust are absolutely essential not only for discipleship but also for the biblical recovery process.

Belief versus Unbelief

As was mentioned in the previous section, John's purpose for writing his Gospel is clearly to help his readers believe in Jesus. It naturally follows that his book would shed much light on the subject of belief.

The word *believe* (*pisteuō*) is used ninety-eight times throughout John's Gospel.[6] Interestingly, this major theme of belief is woven together with the opposite theme of unbelief and provides the stage on which a tension-filled plot is played out. The growing faith of Christ's followers is consistently countered with the growing unbelief of his enemies.

Tenney argues that one of the keys to interpreting John's Gospel is to understand the conflictive interaction between belief and unbelief. He suggests that the belief/unbelief pattern can be clearly seen throughout his book. He has provided a helpful chart that outlines the progressive nature of this conflict:[7]

1. The Prologue: The Proposal for Belief	1:1–18
2. The Presentation for Belief	1:19–4:54
3. The Reactions of Belief and Unbelief	5:1–6:71
4. The Crystallization of Belief and Unbelief	7:1–11:53
5. The Crisis of Belief and Unbelief	11:54–12:50
6. The Assurance for Belief	13:1–17:26
7. The Rejection by Unbelief	18:1–19:42
8. The Vindication of Belief	20:1–31
9. Epilogue: The Dedication of Belief	21:1–25

If the above structuring is an accurate assessment of the development of belief and unbelief in John's Gospel, it unequivocally reveals a black-and-white nature to faith. According to John, either one is a believer or an unbeliever. There can be no gray area when it comes to commitment (or lack of commitment) to Jesus Christ.

In light of this analysis, the events recorded in John necessarily clarify and define the real meaning of belief and unbelief. This is a crucial distinction made by the apostle and is especially important for recovering disciples. Because there seems to be so much confusion in the evangelical church today about the true nature of belief and unbelief, a renewed understanding of John's definition is desperately needed.

A distorted view of belief and unbelief has led many Christians to misunderstand fellow believers who are in emotional pain. Unfortunately, Christians in pain have often been accused of being in a state of *unbelief*. The fact that these believers are depressed and full of emotional turmoil supposedly proves that they lack faith. Their problems are interpreted as being a direct result of unbelief.

Those who have been harshly "diagnosed" by fellow Christians as having a severe case of unbelief know how painful this experience can be. It's like adding insult to injury. Instead of being comforted in their time of need, they find themselves being accused of having a lack of faith.

Is emotional pain and suffering necessarily caused by a lack of faith? Can belief and unbelief truly be defined strictly on an emotional level (e.g., happiness is a sign of belief; sadness is a sign of unbelief)? Thankfully, the apostle John provides answers to these very complicated questions.

As Tenney's structural presentation revealed, the themes of belief and unbelief can be traced throughout John's Gospel. Jesus and his message caused a clear and decisive separation between those who believed and those who didn't. The blossoming faith of the disciples is consistently matched by the growing unbelief of Jesus' enemies.

Interestingly, though, John seems to portray the disciples' faith as not being rock-solid from the beginning (John 6:1–9). On the other hand, the unbelief of his enemies was apparent almost immediately (John 5:16–18).

In light of the apostle John's emphasis, we can come to a crucial conclusion about the true nature of belief and unbelief in his Gospel. True belief, as it is defined by John, is characterized by questioning, faltering, but ultimately following the Lord Jesus (see John 6:5–7, 68; 13:6–9, 38; 14:5, 8–10, 22–24; 20:24–28; 21:1–22). Unbelief, on the other hand, is primarily described as hating, despising, criticizing, and ultimately rejecting the Lord (see John 2:18–20; 5:16–47; 6:41–66; 7:14–44; 8:31–58; 18:1–19:42).

This study of belief and unbelief in the Book of John can assure us that emotional pain and depression are not necessarily a sign of unbelief. Questioning, faltering, doubting, grieving, fearing that God has abandoned you, going through periods when God doesn't make sense are all part of life and an intregal part of the Christian experience. In fact, these trials can actually be a sign that you are growing in the Lord!

One important thing that John does make clear is that a true disciple will always ultimately follow and obey the Lord Jesus. You may go through times when you feel you will ultimately turn away; trials may cause you to fall away for a time, as Peter and the other apostles did (John 18:1–27), but a *true* disciple will always come back.

However, those who consistently disobey and reject the Lord's leading in their lives, who ultimately produce no fruit for his kingdom (John 15), are the ones who are in a state of unbelief. They have a hardened heart and are not to be considered true disciples. In fact, when the veneer is stripped away, they are children of the devil (John 8:42–47).

This black-and-white dimension of John's theology is difficult for us to accept in the American evangelical church today, where gray areas abound in this nonjudgmental age of tolerance. We must resist the pull of popular culture and strive to practice the truths God has revealed to us through John's black-and-white perspective on belief and unbelief. John's clear and helpful guidelines will help us discern between true and false disciples, but they will also keep us from prematurely judging our brothers and sisters in Christ who are not unbelieving but hurting.

For example, Jesus' personal interviews with Nicodemus (John 3) and the Samaritan woman (John 4) keenly demonstrate what true belief is. They are also fascinating studies in regard to discipleship and recovery. Both of them come from completely different social backgrounds (he is a Pharisee and she is a foreigner), and yet important recovery-related issues are evident in both.

Nicodemus and the Samaritan woman both encountered Jesus and were uniquely challenged to believe in him. Initially, they faltered with the truth about him and themselves, but ultimately they believed and followed him. They perfectly fit John's description of true belief. Their discipleship and recovery process can teach us a lot about our own.

Nicodemus

There were some foundational questions burning in the heart of Nicodemus concerning the origins of the Galilean rabbi known as Jesus. He approached Jesus at night, probably because he didn't want the other religious leaders to hear of their conversation. His statements to Jesus would almost certainly have caused his comrades to scorn and ridicule him (John 3:2).

Nicodemus recognized that the signs Jesus was performing proved that he was a teacher sent from God. Jesus, however, was not satisfied with a mere recognition of his divine empowerment. He informed Nicodemus that in order for him to truly understand

and "see the kingdom of God," he must be "born again" (John 3:3). Nicodemus was completely puzzled by Jesus' statement, fully recognizing the physical impossibility involved.

Jesus, however, was not speaking of natural birth at all but of spiritual birth. The transformation of the soul by the Spirit is a profound mystery. Like the blowing of the wind, it is an invisible reality. The effects are clearly visible, but the process itself is unseen (John 3:5–8). The only way for Nicodemus (and us) to truly comprehend the love of God, which was revealed in the giving of his Son, was for him to be spiritually born again (John 3:3, 16).

John did not record Nicodemus's response to Christ's teaching, but it must have had an impact on him. The next time we encounter him is in John 7:50–52, where he is defending Jesus before his fellow Pharisees. Then in John 19:38–39, Nicodemus, along with Joseph of Arimathea, "came out of the closet" and openly admitted their belief in Jesus by burying him.

The truth about Nicodemus was that he was a disciple of Christ, but he was under a tremendous amount of pressure to keep his real identity secret. Nicodemus was trying desperately to be something he wasn't—namely, an unbelieving Pharisee. He was, in essence, living a lie.

Those who come from abusive or dysfunctional backgrounds know what it's like to live a lie. Not only did they have to consistently lie to themselves about the gravity of their situation, but they had to lie to the world in order to save face and keep the family secret intact. The implication from Nicodemus's life is that the truth will eventually come out. Our words and actions will make the truth known sooner or later.

Discipleship and recovery both require a "coming out of the closet" about our situation, regardless of the consequences. Like Nicodemus, we must openly acknowledge our faith in Jesus, the one who has transformed us through spiritual rebirth and given us new, eternal identity as children of God (John 1:12).

The Samaritan Woman

Jesus Christ, who was grace and truth incarnate, is the revealer of all truth concerning God and humanity. He manifests the true nature of God and exposes the deep, dark secrets of the heart. There is no place to hide from the one who came to bring light. This can be a very scary thing to those who have many skeletons in the closet due to a sordid past. They fear his judgment and condemnation.

Thankfully, the account of the Samaritan woman (John 4) can calm the fears of everyone who is ashamed of an awful past. Her story is a beautiful example of how Christ can penetrate a life with both *grace* and *truth*. Like Nicodemus, but to a larger degree, her life story also insightfully reveals the great human capacity to dismiss grace and deny truth.

The scene opens at Jacob's well in Sychar. Jesus was resting by the well when he was suddenly approached by a Samaritan woman coming to draw water. He asked her for a drink, which surprised her because Jews did not associate with Samaritans (John 4:4–9). He in turn offered her "living water," and, like Nicodemus, she did not understand that he was speaking of spiritual, not natural, realities (vv. 10–15).

Then Jesus quickly got to the heart of the matter. His subsequent statements unmistakably unveiled the secrets of her past:

> He said to her, "Go, call your husband, and come here." The woman answered and said, "I have no husband." Jesus said to her, "You have well said, 'I have no husband'; for you have had five husbands, and the one whom you now have is not your husband; this you have said truly."
>
> John 4:16–18

The look on her face must have exposed her embarrassment and shock. So she quickly changed the subject to another topic—the matter of worship. "Our fathers worshiped in this mountain, and you people say that in Jerusalem is the place where men ought to worship" (v. 20).

Jesus revealed to her that the *physical* place of worship is not as important as the *attitude* of the heart: "True worshipers shall worship the Father in spirit and truth; for such people the Father seeks to be His worshipers. God is spirit, and those who worship Him must worship in spirit and truth" (vv. 23–24).

This woman was confronted with more truth that day than she probably ever thought possible! The interesting thing to note is that when the woman went back to town, she did not tell the people about the new spiritual principles for worship. Instead she said, "Come, see a man who told me all the things that I have done; this is not the Christ, is it?" (v. 29).

This is simply amazing. The woman admitted that the Messiah would come and proclaim all things concerning true worship (v. 25). Jesus did reveal to her that he was in fact that Messiah. She seemed to have believed his claim (v. 26). Based on her confession to the townspeople in verse 29, she did not believe because of what Jesus disclosed to her about true worship (although this is very important), but she believed because of what he said concerning her!

It is clear that the Messiah reveals truth about God and also has the ability to search the human heart. For the Samaritan woman it was the latter, not the former, that seemed to have made a believer out of her. Be that as it may, the obvious implication from the entire story is that our relationship with God and our worship of him must be based on truth—truth about God and ourselves.

Another implication is that a sinful and shameful past should not hinder a true belief in God.[8] He accepts all who come to him "in spirit and truth" (John 4:24). Both discipleship and recovery must have truth as their foundation. Truth does not widen the chasm between God and human beings, but it actually closes the gap and brings them together.

Nicodemus and the Samaritan woman were both challenged to faith in Christ. He was a respected and honored Pharisee; she was an outcast and a foreigner, but both of them had obvious problems and needs in their lives. Both of them equally needed to believe in Jesus for salvation, and both of them abundantly received his grace and mercy.

There is little doubt that both of them went through times of trouble—times when they questioned Jesus and faltered in their faith. Yet one thing is certain: If they really believed in Jesus, they would steadfastly follow him to the end. Steadfastness is the mark of true discipleship and should be evident, to some degree, in all believers.

Questioning Faith, Faltering Faith, Following Faith

"'You believe at last!' Jesus answered. 'But a time is coming, and has come, when you will be scattered, each to his own home. You will leave me all alone'" (John 16:31–32 NIV).

It was a time of celebration and revelation. It was a time of intimacy and transparency. It was a time of reflection and introspection. Their time together was coming to an end. Jesus would be leaving soon. He and his disciples had gathered together in the upper room to celebrate his last Passover meal (John 13–16). That is when the Twelve let down their guard and bared their hearts.

Their questions started to pour out like a cascade of water. Peter asked, "Lord, where are You going?" and "Lord, why can I not follow You right now?" (John 13:36–37). Thomas asked, "Lord, we do not know where You are going, how do we know the way?" (John 14:5). Judas (not Iscariot) inquired, "Lord, what then has happened that You are going to disclose Yourself to us, and not to the world?" (John 14:22).

Fear and confusion gripped their hearts at the thought of Jesus leaving them! They had walked with him and learned to trust him, and now he seemed to be deserting them. In fact, Jesus told the disciples it was actually to their advantage that he leave them! If he did not leave, the Holy Spirit would not come. After his departure he would send the Helper, the Holy Spirit (John 16:7).

The coming of the Holy Spirit would mark the beginning of a new and deeper relationship between the disciples, Jesus, and the Father. Jesus was not going to leave them as orphans. Through the Holy Spirit, he and the Father would be with them forever. They would know God more intimately than they ever thought possible. This new relationship would be based on love and obedience:

If you love Me, you will keep My commandments. And I will ask the Father, and He will give you another Helper, that He may be with you forever; that is the Spirit of truth, whom the world cannot receive, because it does not behold Him or know Him, but you know Him because He abides with you, and will be in you. I will not leave you as orphans; I will come to you. After a little while the world will behold Me no more; but you will behold Me; because I live, you shall live also. In that day you shall know that I am in My Father, and you in Me, and I in you. He who has My commandments and keeps them, he it is who loves Me; and he who loves Me shall be loved by My Father, and I will love him, and will disclose Myself to him.

John 14:15–21

The disciples were entering into a new stage in their relationship with Christ. The one they had known and walked with *in the flesh* would now be with them *in the Spirit*. The one they had seen with their eyes would now live in their hearts. They were embarking on a lifelong journey into a world that was completely unknown to them. They were now going to have to live by faith.

This must have been scary for the disciples. They were accustomed to (and probably very comfortable with) seeing Jesus, walking with him, and talking to him face-to-face. Life by faith would be so much more unpredictable and uncontrollable! Yet faith was absolutely necessary to bring them to maturity and produce the spiritual fruit God desired (John 15).

Those first disciples discovered, as have we, that the spiritual life—the life of faith—can be very difficult at times. They quickly learned that the maturing process can be painful! They questioned, they faltered, but ultimately they believed and followed him to the end (John 16:30; Acts 1–2). They eventually learned to walk confidently with their unseen Savior.

We might be tempted to think that this process of faith was easier for the first disciples. After all, they knew Jesus personally. However, as we have seen, their firsthand knowledge of him did not cure their shortsightedness nor free them from the bonds of human weakness. They saw but still went through periods of doubt and confusion (Matt. 28:17; John 16:17–18). Jesus did not reject them because of their weakness but was patient with them as they grew up.

How much more will Jesus accept us who have not had the benefits of seeing as the first disciples did yet have believed anyway! In fact, in his conversation with Thomas, he gives those who have never seen him a special blessing: "Because you have seen Me, have you believed? Blessed are they who did not see, and yet believed" (John 20:29).

Those of us who truly believe, but struggle at times, should be greatly encouraged by the genuine, but sometimes faltering, faith of the disciples and the intimate interaction they had with Jesus the night before he was crucified. It was an atmosphere of acceptance and love meant to encourage struggling disciples in every generation.

Christ's comfort and promises concerning the Holy Spirit unreservedly apply to us in the twentieth century (John 14:23–24; 17:13–26). We who believe in him have been born again by the Spirit and are eternally indwelt by him (John 3:3; 14:16–17). We, like the first disciples, are safe and secure and never have to fear abandonment.

Jesus told us these things so that in him we might have peace. We can experience this peace in the midst of trouble and hardship, knowing that he has overcome the world (John 16:33). We can rest assured that as recovering disciples, true believers who stumble and falter in the faith, we will continue to overcome in him. Christ will help us to conquer the obstacles we face in this life. He will bring us to spiritual freedom and maturity as we continually walk with him by faith.

5

Recovering Disciples, Building Blocks of the Church

Acts of the Apostles

Back in the early 1980s, I had the fascinating opportunity to monitor the progress of the building of a beautiful rock house by a friend in the central Texas hill country. Over several years of living in the area, I had seen quite a number of classic older rock houses, constructed from the rugged rock of the hill country. This, however, was the only one that I got to see go up from the foundation.

What a challenge for the builder! As if fitting together bricks of the same size and shape weren't tough enough, a rock mason has to put all those uniquely shaped natural rock building blocks together as a harmonious whole. Frankly, as I looked at all the irregular shaped rocks lying around near the beginning of that house's construction, I thought there was no way that it would fit together as planned.

I was dead wrong! That rock mason was an artist who understood exactly where to put each unique piece of rock and just how much to reshape it to play its role in the overall house plan. Through my consistent observation, I learned that odd shapes and jagged edges will not stop a skilled mason from completing his task.

The building of such a house made of rock is an apt illustration of how recovery and disciples relate in the Book of Acts. As will be seen, disciples are the building blocks of the church that Jesus had promised to build (Matt. 16:18). Thus, how the individual disciple and groups of disciples relate to the church is a fresh and crucial part of what the New Testament teaches about discipleship.

It must also immediately be noted that many of those brand-new and growing disciples are like irregular pieces of rock, clearly evidencing recovery issues in their lives. In that light, it is quite plausible to infer that the church was intended by the Lord from the beginning to be a setting in which recovery needs were faced and worked through as a foundational part of its ministry.

This chapter will first explore just how influential recovery was in shaping Acts, from its overarching structure to the selection of certain seemingly cameo people or events. Then attention will be turned to distinctive vantage points on discipleship as the means to the end of building the church to the ends of the earth (Acts 1:8).

Recovery as a Framework for the Book of Acts

There seems to be two standard frameworks for outlining the Book of Acts. The first is according to two significant disciples who are successively spotlighted by the author. A Spirit-filled Peter, the great apostle to the Jews (Gal. 2:7–8), stands astride Acts 1–12. Then an equally Spirit-energized Paul, the groundbreaking apostle to the Gentiles (Gal. 2:7–8), is the dominant character in Acts 13–28.[1]

It should be noted that both are mentioned in the other half (in which they are not featured), but only as supporting actors. Paul is seen in Acts 9, 11, and 12, setting the stage for his central role in chapters 13–28. Peter, on the other hand, reemerges only in Acts 15, tying up some of the major theological loose ends left from chapters 1–12 at the Jerusalem council.

When working with this overview outline of Acts, it should be considered that Peter was just recovering from his epic bout with denial (Matt. 26:69–75)[2] as his focal (first) half of the book begins. Similarly, Paul appears to have been virtually a rage-aholic in terms of his intense anger and hatred toward the church (Acts 8:3; 9:1) prior to his conversion on the Damascus Road. That point was undoubtedly considered to be still fresh in the minds of the readers as they came to the latter half of the book in which Paul is the star.

Thus, without proceeding any deeper into the Book of Acts than an overview outline, it is seen that Acts is a book about recovery because it focuses on the lives and ministries of two recovering apostles. However, the other common approach to outlining Acts also yields a related point.

An even more widely used approach to tracking the outline of Acts is according to the geographical progress of the good news, following the outward movement of Acts 1:8—the presumed theme verse of the book. In this case, the Spirit-empowered witness to the Jews is described in chapters 1–7. Then the witness spreads to the rest of Judea and even to the hated Samaritans in chapter 8 (or 8–12 in some outlines). Finally, the gospel witness reaches to the Gentile "dogs," who inhabit the "remotest part of the earth" (1:8) in Acts 9–28 (or 13–28).[3]

Even this geographic-ethnic outline reflects a recovery perspective. The outward spread of the gospel forced the initially totally Jewish church to have to face its astoundingly deep-seated resentment and distrust of both the Samaritans and the Gentiles. As indicated by Peter's stubborn resistance to the divinely given vision (Acts 10–11) and the persistent, enraged persecution that Paul had to face (e.g., chap. 14), the Jews definitely had a lot of recovering to do!

Lower Profiles of Recovery in Acts

Yes, the roles of recovering Peter and Paul provide the broad brush strokes of the structuring of the Book of Acts. It should not be overlooked, however, that recovery also is present in Acts in more subtle hues.

For example, there is the case of Tabitha/Dorcas and the widows in the church in Joppa (Acts 9:36–43).[4] Widows would certainly have to deal with grief and emptiness—both recovery issues. Also, the fact that these widows had to be largely supported by Dorcas (9:39) likely indicates that they were among the destitute needing charity (v. 36) or without any other family to support them—a demeaning and depressing predicament.

Then, there is the situation of John Mark, the helper of Paul and Barnabas on the first missionary journey (13:5), who bailed out and went home (15:36–39). Ironically, Paul, who had earlier been given a great deal of support during a very difficult time by Barnabas (9:26–27), refused to similarly support John Mark. But, again, Barnabas was there to help John Mark pick up the pieces and get on the road to recovery (15:39).[5]

We also should not overlook the demon-possessed woman in Philippi (16:16–18).[6] Though the biblical text does not clearly state that she was converted when the demons were cast out,[7] in all likelihood this is a classic example of recovery from the effects of the occult.

Sadly, there are also blown opportunities for recovery noted in Acts. A short list includes the denial of Ananias and Sapphira (Acts 5), the angry hard-heartedness of all but a few of the Jewish leaders (6:7; cf. 7:51–58), and the self-delusion of almost all of the Greek intellectuals on the Areopagus, who were willing to eagerly consider any new idea but not their own sinful needs (17:19–34).

A Physician with a Heart for Recovering Disciples

There is very strong reason to hold that Dr. Luke, a Gentile, was the author of both the Third Gospel and the Book of Acts.[8] Part of the evidence for that conclusion is that the author was an eyewitness to the so-called "we" passages in Acts (in chaps. 16 and 20–28), which include the recovery of the demon-possessed woman in Philippi. What can be surmised about Luke from elsewhere and strong tradition outside the Bible point to him as the strongest candidate.

A striking angle about this conclusion is that it reflects on Luke as being a physician (Col. 4:14) with a great heart for the needs of people hurting with recovery needs and problems. It is also an invaluable service to the church that he shows that a growing disciple, such as Timothy (Acts 16:1–3), can still be a person who is deeply affected by painful family background issues (v. 1b).[9]

Disciples and the Church in Acts

Turning to the discussion of discipleship in the Book of Acts requires also studying the church. The reason is that the plural *disciples* and *church* become interchangeable in Acts.

By way of analogy, in Acts the term *church* is like focusing on a football team gathered in the huddle. On the other hand, the term *disciples* is like having the focus on the individual members deployed on the line of scrimmage to execute the play (called in the huddle). This frequent, complementary usage in Acts is visualized in table 5.1.

Table 5.1
***Disciples* and *Church:* Interchangeable Terms in Acts**

Mention of *Disciples*	Mention of *Church*	Location
6:1	5:11	Jerusalem
6:7	8:1	Jerusalem
9:1	8:1	Jerusalem
9:38	9:31	Judea (Galilee and Samaria)
11:26	11:26	Syrian Antioch
14:22	14:23	Asia Minor
14:28	14:27	Syrian Antioch
20:30	20:28	Ephesus

The significance of this interchangeability is significant for our study of the rest of the New Testament material: the Epistles and Revelation. The reason is that the term *disciple(s)* is not found in any of those books.[10] However, since the term *church*, and other interchangeable concepts such as *saints* (Acts 9:31, 32, 36, 38, 41) and *Christians* (11:26), are present in force, there is a very real sense in which the idea of discipleship is still alive and well after the Book of Acts.[11]

Five Spotlighted Disciples in Acts

Of the well over 250 uses in the New Testament of the Greek term *mathētēs*, normally translated "disciple(s),"[12] only twenty-eight, or a little over 10 percent, are singular. Of these twenty-eight, the majority (sixteen) refer to the "beloved disciple" in the Gospel of John. The others are found in Luke 6:40; 14:26, 27, 33 (and the parallel passage in Matt. 10:24–25[13]), and the Book of Acts.

This rare, singular usage in Acts seems to point out the five individual disciples who were named as those who embody in various ways the well-known principles of discipleship found in Luke 14:26–33 (i.e., the commitment of carrying the cross and counting the cost).[14] There may be more, however.

It appears that these five instances form a chiasm—a literary pattern that shows parallel thoughts or mirroring ideas in a particular passage of Scripture. This mirroring effect may highlight even more their roles in Luke's plan for the Book of Acts (see table 5.2).

If such a chiastic (inverted parallel) understanding is correct, then three points of significance for discipleship emerge:

1. Ananias and Mnason (Acts 9, 21) are models of the way that wise, long-standing disciples should help other disciples.
2. Saul and Timothy are examples of the fact that even controversial, younger disciples are worth the calculated risk (Acts 9, 16).
3. Even though "female disciple" is found only once in the New Testament, it is more than a merely casual usage.[15]

As the focus of the chiastic structure, Dorcas (and, by implication, other female disciples) is honored as a very significant disciple indeed!

Carrying Out the Great Commission in Acts

It is quite possible that Luke had access to the Gospel of Matthew when he carefully researched and composed the Book of Acts (see Luke 1:1–4), though that is by no means certain. If not, Luke surely possessed most of the same source material that

Table 5.2
The Singular of *Disciple* in Acts

Passage	Person / Key Data	Place
9:10	A. Ananias, a veteran disciple who aids newly converted Saul (Paul)	Damascus
9:26	B. Saul (Paul), a controversial, newer disciple because of his background (persecuting the church)	Jerusalem
9:36	C. Tabitha/Dorcas, the only specifically stated female disciple (*Greek mathetria*) in the New Testament	Joppa
16:1	B[1]. Timothy, a controversial, newer disciple because of his (mixed ethnic) background*	Central Asia Minor
21:16	A[1]. Mnason, a veteran disciple who aids the apostle Paul	En route to Jerusalem

*For a more in-depth discussion of the discipleship of Timothy, especially in relationship to the role of his mother, see "Discipleship in a Mixed Marriage: Eunice," chapter 12 in Luter and McReynolds, *Women as Christ's Disciples*.

Matthew had because of the parallels in the First and Third Gospels that are not present in Mark.[16]

This point is important to establish because it makes it almost a given that Luke was fully aware of the version of the Great Commission found at the end of Matthew's Gospel. If so, it can be no accident that the spread of the gospel and the church in Acts takes place over and over again by the three-step disciple-making process mandated by the risen Lord in Matthew 28:19–20:

1. *going* evangelistically (v. 19)
2. *baptizing* the converts (v. 19)
3. *teaching* the new disciples to progress to full obedience to the Lord (v. 20)

Table 5.3 shows just how consistently these three steps keep popping up at each new forward movement of the gospel witness in Acts.

As stated earlier, this pattern of repetition is much too extensive to be coincidental. Rather, it is a clear indicator that the apostles (and Luke) took very seriously their commission to "make disciples of all the nations . . . even to the end of the age" (Matt. 28:19–20).[17]

Recovery and Discipleship Together in the Church

As has been seen in Acts, the church that Jesus Christ is building (Matt. 16:18) was never designed by the Lord to be a new car showroom! Unlike a car dealership, which flaunts its new product as being shiny and perfect, it is not realistic to expect new believers to be fully mature disciples from the beginning (even though that impression is left by false expectations in certain churches).

No, the church is supposed to be a paint and body shop, in which the marring scrapes and dents haunting the lives of Christ's disciples are repaired.[18] It was divinely designed to be a spiritual hospital in which emotionally and relationally hurting disciples are in a context to get well and keep growing. It is also a spiritual/emotional HMO (health maintenance organization) for those who, by the Lord's grace, either are not beset by such problems or who already have worked through them to a substantial degree. Those kinds of persons are able to grow as full-speed-ahead disciples.

Thus, it seems fair to say that the church that is seen being born and growing in the Book of Acts was the original Christian support group.[19] If we take seriously what we observe in Acts, we will be deeply impacted by the early church's example of meeting needs within the context of unified, supportive fellowship (e.g., Acts 2:42–47).

Table 5.3
The Disciple-Making Commission
(Matthew 28:19–20)
Fulfilled in Acts*

Setting/hearers	Pentecost	Samaria	Ethiopian eunuch	Cornelius's group (Gentiles)	Syrian Antioch	Asia Minor (first missionary journey)	Philippi (second missionary journey)	Corinth (second missionary journey)	Ephesus (third missionary journey)
Make Disciples!						Acts 14:21 (only use outside Matthew)			
Going/ evangelism	2:38	8:5, 12	8:35	10:43	11:20, 21, 24	14:21a	16:14, 30, 32	18:4, 4, 8a	19:2, 4, 10
Baptizing	2:41	8:12b, 13, 16	8:36, 38	10:47–48a			16:15, 33	18:8b	19:5
Teaching	2:42			10:48	11:23, 26	14:22 (16:15; 18:23)	(20:2)	18:11 (20:3)	19:9–10 (20:27, 31)

*The seminal thinking behind this chart was developed by A. Boyd Luter, *A New Testament Theology of Discipling* (Dallas: Dallas Theology Seminary, 1985); and A. Boyd Luter, "Great Commission," in *Anchor Bible Dictionary*, ed. David Noel Freedman (Garden City, N.Y.: Doubleday, 1992), 2:1090–91.

It is in just such an environment that disciples can "bear one another's burdens" (Gal. 6:2) and "rejoice with those who rejoice, and weep with those who weep" (Rom. 12:15), as Paul, the hero of the second half of Acts, directed his readers to do. If that doesn't make for an optimally healthy, sensitive, supportive group, what does?

6

Spiritual Freedom and Recovery

Romans and Galatians

I was seized with the conviction that I must understand [Paul's] letter to the Romans . . . but to that moment one phrase in chapter 1 stood in my way. I hated the idea, "in it the righteousness of God is revealed." . . . I hated the righteous God who punishes sinners. . . .

At last, meditating day and night and by the mercy of God, I . . . began to understand that the righteousness of God is that through which the righteous live by a gift of God, namely by faith. . . . Here I felt as if I were entirely born again and had entered paradise itself through gates that had been flung open.

Martin Luther

In a very real sense, the Protestant Reformation was born out of one man's intense personal struggles. Martin Luther was a man deeply troubled by his conscience. Though he was a rigorously devoted Augustinian monk, he felt he could not measure up to God's holy standards.

No matter how many times he confessed his sins and repented, he was convinced that his meager efforts were not enough to appease an angry, righteous God. Luther's faithful friend and superior, Johann von Staupitz, tried to calm his doubts by assuring him that he was forgiven. But the young Luther found no comfort: "Yet my conscience would never give me assurance, but I was always doubting and said, 'You did not perform that correctly. You were not contrite enough. You left that out of your confession.'"[1]

Eventually, after a long period of study and meditation, the Scriptures were opened to Luther, and his heart was set free. He finally understood from the Book of Romans, Galatians, and others the grace, mercy, and righteousness of God. He realized that the righteous please God by faith, not by works.

With this astounding revelation, his veil of doubt was ripped away. Luther was released from bondage and experienced true joy and spiritual freedom. His biblical discoveries shaped the Protestant Reformation and have influenced countless thousands of believers over the past five centuries.

Many believers in recovery can readily identify with Luther's intense personal struggles and feelings of inadequacy. They can also, all too easily, identify with his fear of the wrath of God. Unlike Luther, however, they have yet to experience release from bondage. They do not yet know the joy of true spiritual freedom.

For Luther, spiritual freedom was realized when he understood from his study of the Scriptures—the Books of Romans and Galatians in particular—that he was not in bondage to the law. He discovered that a person is justified (declared not guilty), not by works of the law, but by faith in Jesus Christ.

Those who believe in Jesus Christ have received the Spirit of God and live according to the standards of the Spirit. They are not in bondage to the flesh (that is, the law), but they are controlled by the Spirit of God. As Martin Luther discovered, true spiritual liberty is found in understanding these crucial scriptural truths.

In light of this, it is of utmost importance that we understand the apostle Paul's flesh/Spirit concepts in Romans and Galatians. Perhaps there are no two theological concepts more misunderstood or misinterpreted than that of the flesh and the Spirit. How we view discipleship and biblical recovery is directly related to what we believe about the flesh/Spirit concepts.

For the purposes of this chapter, we will focus primarily on Romans 7–8 and Galatians 5–6, which discuss at length the concepts of the flesh and the Spirit. Before we delve specifically into these chapters, however, it is vital that we explore the background and overall purpose of Romans and Galatians. These key chapters must not be lifted out of their original settings but must be understood within the overall contexts of the letters.

The Background and Purpose of Romans and Galatians

There is some debate concerning Paul's purpose in writing the systematic and theologically profound Epistle to the Romans. Many scholars believe that Paul intended to have the Roman church be a base of missionary operation for the West, as the church of Antioch was for the East (Rom. 15:22–24).[2]

Therefore, in order to prepare them for his coming, Paul set forth a complete exposition of the Gospel. It was important that he do this, because he had not yet made a personal visit to the Roman church. Sending the letter ahead of him gave the church ample time to absorb his message and be ready to help him in his missionary endeavors.

This could certainly have been part of the reason why he wrote this epistle, but the apostle seemed to be more concerned about apparent conflicts between certain members of the Roman congregation. The church at Rome was comprised of both Jews and Gentiles. This is obvious by Paul's many references to both people groups throughout his letter (e.g., Rom. 1:16; 2:9–10; 3:9; 4:16–17).

The church there had recently gone through a lot of changes. Claudius had expelled all Jews from Rome. This would have naturally included all Christian Jews, like Priscilla and Aquila (Acts 18:2). The situation would have forced the Gentile Christians who were left behind to completely reorganize themselves.

The synagogues, where Gentile believers gathered with their Jewish Christian brothers, were all closed due to the Claudius edict. This brought about the development of house churches. Wiefel gives extraordinary insight into this historical situation:

Creation of these semi-legal house churches eliminated the Jewish element which previously had been rooted in the synagogue assembly. This explains why Jewish Christianity did not regain its dominant position and why Paul, in his letter to the Romans, assumed that his readers were those who lived by the gospel of freedom from the law. Accordingly, the Jewish-Christians, who probably returned in great numbers only after the Claudius edict was finally repealed, found a "new" Christian congregation completely different in organizational structure and spiritual outlook from the old one which had existed in the synagogue. Now they are only a minority in a congregation which previously they had shaped. From this emerges the possibility of specifying the [purpose] of Romans: it was written to assist the Gentile Christian majority, who are the primary addressees of the letter, to live together with the Jewish Christians in one congregation, thereby putting an end to their quarrels about status.[3]

It is perhaps feasible to assume that the "weak" referred to in Romans 14:1–15:13 are the Jewish Christians who returned to Rome. However, Paul's attempt to bring unity and harmony between Jew and Gentile is relatively clear throughout the letter. It is against this backdrop of the Jew/Gentile controversy that we must understand Romans 7–8.

The churches at Galatia also faced a Jew/Gentile problem, but one of a different nature than that at Rome. The Galatian churches were comprised of primarily Gentile believers, though there were quite a few Jews who had been converted. Paul preached the gospel to them on his first missionary journey, and the churches became well established (Acts 14).

Not long after that, some conservative Jews, known as Judaizers or legalizers, came to Galatia and claimed that in order for the Gentiles to be saved, they must be circumcised and keep the law of Moses (see Acts 15). This was in direct contradiction to what the apostle Paul had previously taught them.

Nevertheless, some of the Galatian Christians believed the Judaizers and were turning to the law and circumcision (Gal. 5:1–12). This is what prompted Paul to write the Galatian epistle. Boice comments:

Paul was immediately filled with righteous indignation. He saw in a moment that if the views of the legalizers prevailed, grace and the cross of Jesus Christ would be emptied of all value (5:2–4). Moreover, Christianity would lose its distinctive character and soon become little more than a minor sect of Judaism. In righteous anger, Paul wrote this letter to reprove legalism and regain the Galatian churches.[4]

Paul's poignant discussion of the flesh and the Spirit in Galatians 5:13–26 must be seen in the light of his conflict with the Judaizers and his defense of the true gospel. This crucial passage is sandwiched between Paul's discourse on the inadequacies of circumcision of the flesh and of the law (5:1–12; 6:11–18). This must be taken into consideration when interpreting the text.

The Flesh and the Spirit: Two Views

There are two very important key questions we want to explore concerning the concepts of the flesh and the Spirit in Romans and Galatians: Should we understand the flesh/Spirit antithesis in Paul's writings to mean that Christians have two natures, a "sinful" one and a "new" one, that are at odds with one another? Or should we understand the flesh/Spirit antithesis to represent two historical eras, separated by the death and resurrection of Jesus Christ?

To put it another way, do the flesh/Spirit passages describe an internal, psychological and spiritual battle of two natures within the Christian? Or do they describe a historical *pre* (in the flesh) and *post* (in the Spirit) conversion existence? How we interpret these key passages has a direct bearing on the discipleship and recovery process.

For example, if Paul is speaking about an inner duality, then it would seem that we are doomed to a Jekyll-and-Hyde Christian existence. We could actually be in the flesh one minute and in the Spirit the next. It does not seem, in this case, that consistent Christian living is a realistically obtainable goal.

If, on the other hand, Paul is talking about two historical eras, then a true Christian is always in the Spirit. The Christian life is not characterized by a flesh/Spirit existence. Those who are believers in Christ are historically and consistently in the Spirit. In this case, mature (not perfect) Christian living is a reachable goal.

For many of us, our personal experience would dictate that the former interpretation of the flesh/Spirit antithesis is the correct one. Our Christian life has often been a Jekyll-and-Hyde experience. Sometimes we are victorious in our battle against sin. Sometimes we are not. And we generally attribute our success or failure to being in the Spirit or in the flesh.

There is a major practical problem with this view of the flesh and the Spirit. It puts us in a no-win situation. It seems that we are at the mercy of these two natures that battle within us. It also seems that neither we nor God can control the endless war.

"Within this clash Christians have been graphically portrayed as cages that contain both the black dog of the old nature and the white dog of the new nature."[5] These two "dogs" are constantly fighting to gain control. The one who wins will determine our behavior.

Where, then, is the Christian freedom the apostle Paul talks about in these same flesh/Spirit passages (Rom. 8:1–3; Gal. 5:13)? We do not experience it because we see ourselves as being held captive by two opposing natures! Unfortunately, this view gives us an opportunity to theologize our sinful failures. In it, we find a way to shuck responsibility for our actions.

The inner duality view of the flesh and the Spirit has apparently been around since the time of Augustine. Yet theologians down through the centuries, and especially in recent years, have questioned this interpretation.[6] They favor the redemptive-historical view of the flesh and Spirit.

These scholars also believe these important flesh/Spirit passages have been misunderstood primarily because the immediate and overall contexts of the passages have been virtually ignored. We tend to agree with these scholars that the redemptive-historical view of the flesh and Spirit is much more in line with Paul's thinking.

As Walt Russell has suggested, we need a new set of interpretative glasses, a pair that corresponds more closely to Paul's set of glasses.[7] The redemptive-historical understanding of the flesh/Spirit passages can positively impact the discipleship and recovery process. It is our goal to present this perspective to you as clearly as possible.

Ridderbos discusses at length the redemptive-historical view of the flesh and Spirit in Paul's writings and shows how he relates them directly back to the person and work of Christ:

"Flesh" and "Spirit" represent two modes of existence, on the one hand that of the old aeon which is characterized and determined by the flesh, on the other that of the new creation which is of the Spirit of God. . . . The contrast is therefore of a redemptive-historical nature. . . . It is within this redemptive-historical contrast of flesh and Spirit as the mode of existence of the old and new creation that Paul now views the life of Christ before and after his resurrection. . . . It is in that new existence of the resurrection and of the Spirit, that the church may now know Christ . . . and may also judge itself as joined with him. . . . For this reason the church is no longer "in the flesh," i.e., subject to the regime of the first aeon and the evil powers reigning in it, but "in the Spirit," brought under dominion of freedom in Christ.[8]

According to Ridderbos, then, Paul's concepts of the flesh and Spirit are rooted and grounded in the person and work of Christ. Having laid a general foundation of the flesh/Spirit antithesis from a redemptive-historical perspective, we are now ready to examine them in the context of Romans 7–8 and Galatians 5–6.

Romans 7–8

According to Walt Russell, "Paul uses *flesh* and *Spirit* in antithesis in his extended discussions of the relationship between Jews and Gentiles in the church in Galatians 3–6, Romans 7–8, and Philippians 3. In these contexts, *flesh* is in tandem with *nomos* ('law') and is associated with the era of Israel under the Mosaic Law."[9]

Paul began his discourse in Romans 7 with the phrase, "for I am speaking to those who know the law" (v. 1), alerting his Jewish audience that he was speaking specifically to them. The Gentiles, though they were not completely exempt from the law (Rom. 3:19–20), were not considered "under the law" as the Jews were.

The fact that Torah (the Law) was a special gift to Israel is made clear in several other passages (Rom. 3:2; 9:4; Eph. 2:11–18). Therefore, it is fair to say that Paul's discussion in Romans 7 holds special significance for the Jews. In verses 4–6, he gave an illustration from marriage to show his Jewish brethren that they have been freed from the law:

Therefore, my brethren, you also were made to die to the Law
through the body of Christ, that you might be joined to another,
to Him who was raised from the dead, that we might bear fruit for
God. For while we were in the flesh, the sinful passions, which were
aroused by the Law, were at work in the members of our body to
bear fruit for death. But now we have been released from the Law,
having died to that by which we were bound, so that we serve in
newness of the Spirit and not in oldness of the letter.

Romans 7:4–6

This must have been quite a revelation to the Jews, who were
so accustomed to restraining immoral behavior through the law.
The Jews needed to hear this from the apostle Paul, who was a
Jew himself, and not from the Gentile Christians who now dominated the Roman church.

What makes verses 7–25 so powerful is that the apostle Paul,
speaking directly to the Jews, brilliantly showed the inadequacies
of the law to restrain immoral behavior. He did this by personi-
fying Israel's experience at Sinai in verses 7–13 and by confessing
his personal experience as a pious Jew under the law in verses
14–25. Moo gives further insight into this interpretation:

Paul's clear tendency to view *nomos* [law] as a special gift to Israel
stands against any "universalistic" interpretation of Rom. 7:7–12.
. . . It seems best, then, to restrict the signification of *nomos/entole*
[law/command] in Rom. 7:7–12 to that body of divine revelation
which had its origin with Moses and found its *telos* [end] in Christ
(Rom. 10:4). Such a restriction effectively rules out the (purely)
Adamic view as well as the interpretation which applies Paul's discussion to humankind generally. . . .

In vv. 7–12, then, it seems best to conclude that Paul describes
the experience of Israel at Sinai but uses the first person because he
himself, as a Jew, has been affected by that experience. In vv. 14–25,
where the subsequent struggle of Israel under the law is depicted,
Paul writes with more subjectivity because the struggle is one that
he has to some extent personally experienced. Its ability to explain
the perplexing combination of objective narrative and subjective
confession in Romans 7 is a further strength of the view which has
been presented.[10]

Romans 8, in light of this understanding of Romans 7, also takes on a deeper, more powerful meaning. Because Jewish (and Gentile) believers are now in the Spirit—that is, joined to Christ—they are free from the condemnation of the law (8:1). They are no longer enslaved by the fear of judgment the law brought, but they have been permanently adopted into the family of God (8:15)!

Therefore, what is represented in Romans 7–8 is two historical eras: the old era of the flesh/law and the new era of the Spirit/-Christ. We Gentile believers, who have been grafted into the cultivated olive tree (Rom. 11:11–24), also belong to the new era of the Spirit.

For many of us, to view Romans 7–8 from this historical perspective requires a paradigm shift of epic proportion! After all, the prevailing view among evangelicals is that Paul is describing the Christian experience in Romans 7 and is teaching that believers possess two natures.

However, when the immediate context and overall purpose of the epistle is taken into account, that interpretation does not seem to fit. The reason why the inner duality view is so popular is probably because our daily struggles *seem* to testify to its reality.

While it is true that we will continue to struggle with sin as long as we are in this present state, it does not necessarily mean that it's because we have two opposing natures. Rather, it is because discipleship (and recovery) is a process, and, to be quite frank, many of us are spiritually immature. We are not purposefully seeking to grow up spiritually.

By God's help, we must continually grow in the Spirit and mature in the image of Christ (Rom. 8:29). This is accomplished primarily by studying God's Word, by prayer, by meaningful fellowship with other believers (Acts 2:42–46), and by seeking biblical counsel to help us with our recovery-related issues. The more we "by the Spirit . . . put to death the misdeeds of the body" (Rom. 8:13 NIV) and the more we embrace our new self in Christ (see Rom. 9), the less intense our struggle against sin will become.

The redemptive-historical view of Romans 7–8 can bring us great comfort and assurance. There is abundant peace in knowing that, no matter what we're going through, we are:

1. always in the Spirit (Rom. 8:1–3)
2. always free from judgment and condemnation (Rom. 8:1, 15)
3. always a child of God (Rom. 8:14)
4. always comforted by hope (Rom. 8:24)
5. always more than conquerors through him who loved us (Rom. 8:37)
6. never separated from the love of God (Rom. 8:39)

No, the Christian life was never intended to be a Jekyll-and-Hyde experience. Rather, it was meant to be a life characterized by spiritual strength, peace, hope, and love.

Galatians 5–6

Galatians 5–6 must be understood in the overall context of Paul's conflict with the Judaizers. They claimed to have the true gospel, which made circumcision and observance of Torah necessary for salvation. This brought the apostle Paul into sharp dispute with them, which prompted him to write his letter to the Galatians.

As was pointed out earlier, the key passage (Gal. 5:13–26) is sandwiched between discourses on the inadequacies of circumcision and Torah to restrain immoral behavior. Therefore, Galatians 5–6 is the climax of the apostle's argument against the Judaizers.

In this crucial section, Paul seeks to answer this burning question: Which gospel (his or the Judaizers') gives release from sin's power and manifests true spiritual freedom? By contrasting the behavioral patterns of the two communities of God's people (5:13–26), those who are of the *flesh* and those who are of the *Spirit,* the apostle brilliantly shows that his is the true gospel of spiritual freedom.

Walt Russell summarizes Paul's argument in this way:

> In Paul's framework *flesh* now represents not only the Judaizers' emphasis on their covenant in the flesh with Abraham (Gen. 17:13 LXX), but tragically also all the moral frailty and weakness that characterizes persons on their own, unaided by God's Spirit.
> In this sense, I believe that *flesh* and *Spirit* have become abbreviations in Paul's argument, representing the two competing identities for the people of God in Galatia. The "flesh community"

(Judaizers) is a community identified with the Mosaic law era, and therefore is a community identified and characterized by the frailty and transitoriness of bodily existence and the absence of God's Spirit. . . . By contrast, the "Spirit community" is a community identified and characterized by the presence of God's Spirit and liberation from sin's dominion in the midst of bodily existence.[11]

Similar to our observation in Romans 7–8, Galatians 5–6 is *not* teaching that the Christian vacillates between the flesh and the Spirit. The Christian is in Christ and has entered into the new historical era of the Spirit: "Now those who belong to Christ Jesus have crucified the flesh with its passions and desires" (Gal. 5:24).

Oftentimes, however, we do not feel like we're in the Spirit. The works of the flesh (vv. 19–21) seem to so overtake us that it feels like our flesh and the Spirit are striving against one another, so that we don't do as we really please (v. 17).[12] Sometimes, it feels like the Spirit is actually being swallowed up by our flesh!

We must remember, though, that our identity as people of the Spirit does not change with the battle. We are always people in the Spirit and empowered by the Spirit. Therefore, victory over sinful desires is assured as long as we cooperate with the Spirit. Discipleship and recovery is a maturing process in which the "fruit of the Spirit" (5:22–23) becomes increasingly manifest in our lives as we grow in the grace and knowledge of our Lord.

Russell concludes that the Christian "does not have 'flesh' in Galatians 5:13–26. Instead, the Christian has the true identity mark of the children of Abraham (3:6–14) and the antithetical bodily condition to the flesh (3:1–5). The Christian has the Holy Spirit, not the flesh. Certainly no internal duality exists between these antithetical modes of existence."[13]

In conclusion, true spiritual freedom is found in recognizing our identity as people consistently and historically in the Spirit. That means that the more we mature in the discipleship and recovery process, the less we will be dominated by sinful desires.

7

Confronting Chronic Immaturity

1–2 Corinthians

It hasn't been that many years since a trip to a city like New Orleans or San Francisco was considered to be very much "a walk on the wild side." At that point, certain kinds of immoral and illicit behavior were flaunted only in a handful of locations.

Things change, however. No, I do not mean that "the Big Easy" or Frisco have notably cleaned up their acts (though that may be true to a small extent). Rather, my point is that so many other American cities have become much more like the sleazy, if not shocking, reputations formerly owned by New Orleans and San Francisco.

To coin a term, this "Orleans-izing" (or "Frisco-izing") of the broader American culture is a trend that is also related to certain behavioral patterns. It is hard to get around the conclusion that the patterns in question reflect a pervasive immaturity.

Think about it! What kind of persons are prone to taking undue risks without considering the consequences? What type of people characteristically act in a clearly irresponsible manner (and often seem proud of it)?

There may be more answers than one to this pop quiz. But one answer that cannot be dodged would have to be those whose immature actions emerge from immature emotions and attitudes.

No, I am not picking on the young and relatively inexperienced. If anything, their immaturity is to be expected to one degree or another. However, that is not the situation with the "older, but *not* wiser." Sadly, their additional experience hasn't made much of a difference in terms of growing up, both down deep and behaviorally.

A Challenging Environment for Recovery and Discipleship

The history of the city of Corinth reveals it to be a sort of New Orleans or San Francisco for Achaia (Southern Greece). Prior to the destruction of Corinth by the Romans in 146 B.C., the city had an astoundingly debauched reputation. Out of that era, the verb *to Corinthianize* was created as a synonym for *to fornicate*. Likewise, *Corinthian girl* was widely used to speak of a whore.[1]

Corinth was rebuilt by the Romans in 44 B.C. It is highly doubtful whether it ever again approached the absolutely extreme level of immoral (even by ancient Greek standards) behavior of old Corinth, though that certainly does not mean things had changed completely, either.[2]

Actually, one major related external change had taken place. In the century between the destruction of old Corinth and the rebuilding of new Corinth, the behavioral standards of virtually all the major seaports around the Mediterranean basin had dropped considerably. That trend continued unabated through the New Testament period.

So, it is highly doubtful whether Corinth was the unrivaled cesspool of the first century A.D., as it clearly had been of an earlier era. Suffice it to say that the city that the apostle Paul had ministered in for at least a year and a half at an earlier point was easily still gross enough in its behavior to provide the most likely impetus for the description in Romans 1:18–32.[3] In other words,

Paul's depiction of the tragic end to which unbelieving mankind's unchecked lusts (v. 24) and degrading passions will take them is right off the streets of the Corinth of his day.

Sounds like a tough place to persuade people to become disciples of Jesus Christ and enter full biblical recovery! But that's only part of the context. Hang on and you'll begin to realize just how difficult was the challenge Paul took on in planting a church in Corinth.

The other related, tough-nut-to-crack part of Corinth in that day was its cosmopolitan sophistication linked with its utter fascination with the prevalent Greek philosophy and rhetoric: the Sophists.[4] Much like the media-saturated culture of the late twentieth century, Corinthians loved to be entertained by great rhetoric and fancied themselves as philosophically wise (1 Cor. 1:21–22; 2:4–5).

So there is the blend that existed in Corinth: an appetite for out-of-bounds behavior linked with a candy coating of the rhetorical/philosophical. What does it add up to? What I call "sneaky immaturity": looking mature on the outside because of intelligence and education, but remaining very immature at the emotional core of your being. Many of the people Paul was working with in Corinth—and many people today, including not a few Christians—fit this profile to a T.

Paul's Patience

Just how difficult and demanding was it for the apostle to deal with the largely intelligent, but immature, Corinthian church? One of the best ways to grasp that challenge and Paul's wonderful, Spirit-led patience and self-control (Gal. 5:22–23) is to quickly survey the amazing extent of his interaction with the Corinthians over a period of a very few years.[5] See table 7.1.

Wow! Talk about going the second mile! Paul's relationship with the immature Corinthian disciples was more like a marathon. We will gain more insight about the problem(s) with the Corinthians and the treatment Paul determined that he should utilize by briefly analyzing the structure of both Corinthian letters.

Table 7.1
Paul's "Back-and-Forth" with the Corinthian Church

Event	Scripture
Founding of the church in Corinth (on Paul's second missionary trip)	Acts 18:1–17
Leaving Corinth, arriving at Ephesus	Acts 18:18–19
Writing a letter that is now lost	1 Cor. 5:9–13
Receiving a troubling report from Chloe's household as well as a letter from Corinth	1 Cor. 1:11; 7:1
Writing the letter that is now called 1 Corinthians	1 Corinthians
Sending Timothy and Erastus to Corinth	Acts 19:22; 1 Cor. 4:17; 16:10
Hearing of crisis in Corinth caused by Jews questioning Paul's authority	2 Cor. 10:10; 11:23; 12:6–7
Making a hasty, painful visit to Corinth Writing a severe letter to the Corinthian church	2 Cor. 2:1; 12:14; 13:1 2 Cor. 2:3–9; 7:8–12
Searching for Titus in Troas and Macedonia	2 Cor. 2:12–13
Finding Titus, who reports improvement in Corinth	2 Cor. 7:6–16
Writing the letter that is now called 2 Corinthians	2 Corinthians
Making a third visit to Corinth	Acts 19:21; 20:3; 2 Cor. 13:1

Adapted from H. Wayne House, *Chronological and Background Charts of the New Testament* (Grand Rapids: Zondervan, 1983).

A Framework Understanding of 1 Corinthians

In a basic sense, the structure of 1 Corinthians is an exercise in simple clarity. Essentially, the foundational skeleton for the whole letter is provided by: (1) the mention in 1 Corinthians 1:11 of information Paul had obtained from "Chloe's people"; and (2) the reference in 7:1 to some sort of letter from the Corinthian church, apparently containing a number of questions carried to Paul by a trio from the congregation named in 16:17.[6]

The resulting bare-bones outline looks like this:

I. Reply to disturbing reports about the Corinthian disciples: Stop your worldly, immature behavior! (chaps. 1–6)
II. Reply to various questions from the Corinthian disciples: Change your immature, unscriptural outlooks that lead to false practice and belief! (chaps. 7–16)

Despite the basic accuracy of this approach, that is not all that needs to be known about the structure of 1 Corinthians for the purposes of this study. More recent studies have concluded that, in 1 Corinthians, Paul skillfully employed the most basic chiastic (inverted parallel) structuring in a skillful manner.[7]

Two such examples have clear ramifications here. The first encompasses 1 Corinthians 1:10–3:23 and is laid out by the apostle in the following manner:

A. (1:10–2:5) The wise "foolishness" of the cross versus the foolish wisdom of the world
B. (2:6–16) The Spirit-given wisdom of God, which the world cannot understand
A[1]. (3:1–23) The problem of the Corinthian disciples' worldly, immature ("carnal") behavior

Paul's point in this arrangement is to show his readers that they should not still be following the foolish, unwise ways of the world, especially since they possess the Holy Spirit, who enables spiritual discernment (2:14–16).

The second basic chiastic structure that is key for our understanding of Paul's approach is in chapters 12–14, the well-known "spiritual gifts" passage. It is set up in this way:

- A. (12:1–31) The role of spiritual gifts in the body of Christ: promoting selfless unity through functional diversity
  - B. (13:1–13) The necessary spiritual dynamic energizing spiritual gifts: mature love
- A¹. (14:1–40) The mature usage of spiritual gifts in the worship assembly: selflessly respecting necessary guidelines so all may be edified

In this case, what appears to be the most gifted church seen in the New Testament (1:7) apparently had a prideful fixation on certain spectacular, out-front gifts. Paul lays out chapters 12–14 to counter that immature imbalance: He mirrors the divinely intended purpose of the gifts (chap. 12) and their proper employment in the assembly (chap. 14), while emphasizing that even such impressive gifts are ultimately worthless unless they are prompted by love (chap. 13).

So even this quick look at structural factors in 1 Corinthians is sufficient to demonstrate how engrained was the problem of chronic immaturity that Paul had to take on. Hopefully, things would get better in 2 Corinthians.

A Framework Understanding of 2 Corinthians

Unfortunately, the tone of 2 Corinthians is as much Paul having to explain his actions to the immature Corinthian disciples as him challenging their unwise perspectives and actions. A basic sectional outline of 2 Corinthians might be constructed with the following common four-point breakdown:[8]

- I. Paul discusses the pure motives behind his recent actions (1:1–2:13)
- II. Paul anchors his ministry in the nature of the new covenant (2:14–7:16)
- III. Paul reminds the immature Corinthian disciples of the need for a generous, grateful response to God's uniquely generous grace (8:1–9:15)

IV. Paul defends his apostolic authority in the wake of a recent fixation by the Corinthian church on Jewish false teachers (10:1–13:13)[9]

By this, it is clear that the immature Corinthians were at it again. Fortunately, the apostle was still on the job. There is also good reason to believe that he was continuing his elegant literary confrontation of the problems.

Recently, Craig Blomberg has made a strong case for the following chiastic structuring of 2 Corinthians 1–7.[10]

A. (1:12–22) The Corinthians can rightfully boast in Paul
   B. (1:23–2:11) Grief and comfort over the painful letter; hope for forgiving the offender
      C. (2:12–13) Looking for Titus in Macedonia
         D. (2:14–4:6) Contrasts: belief versus unbelief, centered on Christians as the "letters" of the living God, in glory being transformed into his image
            E. (4:7–5:10) Surviving and triumphing despite every hardship
               F. (5:11–21) The ministry of reconciliation
            E^1. (6:1–10) Surviving and triumphing despite every hardship
         D^1. (6:11–7:4) Contrasts: belief versus unbelief, centered on Christians as the temple of the living God, in light of being transformed into his holiness
      C^1. (7:5–7) Finding Titus in Macedonia
   B^1. (7:8–13a) Grief and comfort over the painful letter; joy after forgiving the offender
A^1. (7:13b–16) Paul can rightfully boast in the Corinthians

This beautiful structure reflects Paul's desire to serve as a model of mature, straightforward communication with his immature Corinthians. Besides dealing with key maturity issues such as forgiveness, consistent faith and spiritual transformation, and perseverance in suffering, the chiasm focuses on a crucial point: reconciliation (5:11–21).

Though Paul's discussion has great theological ramifications for the point at which an individual becomes a Christian, it is not limited to the starting point. Since Paul addresses his readers as "beloved" (7:1) and "brethren" (8:1), he believes they are already reconciled to God in that sense. Instead, he urges on his immature readers (5:20) the need for broader reconciliation in getting past their immature fixation on outward (fleshly) appearances (5:12–17), a typical (and potentially disastrous) shortcoming of immature personalities.

What a powerful point to develop in such an appropriate literary package! In fact, this truth and several other crucial both-sides-of-the-coin lessons about spiritual/emotional maturity (and the lack of same) need to be succinctly etched in stone before concluding this chapter.

Lingering Lesson I

Spiritual immaturity values impressive words or appearances. Whether it be worldly wisdom (as in 1 Cor.) or false apostolic teaching (2 Cor. 10–11), immature people are impressed way too much with the outer trappings and slick presentation.[11] Paul, like the Lord, was much more concerned with the things of the heart (see 1 Sam. 16:7).

Disciples of Christ in any day and time, especially those in recovery, must learn not to place the priority on the outer shell of appearance and image. That is particularly useful advice in a society like ours, which continually hawks its products with cynical adages such as, "Image is everything."

Lingering Lesson II

Spiritual immaturity glorifies prideful giftedness. If anything, this point hits even closer to home in the American evangelical sector in the mid-1990s. By virtue of rapidly growing, glamorous megaministries, flawlessly edited tape ministries, and slick best-selling books, there has come to be a dangerous virtual worshiping of certain golden-tongued preachers and supremely gifted leaders among conservative Christians, much like in Corinth.

Now, most such ministries would immediately disavow any similarity between what they are fostering and the attitudes of the immature Corinthian disciples. Yet many of them were started by a strikingly articulate and charismatic leader, and the whole ministry is built around him and his extraordinary gifts.

So we must ask: To what extent is the constant lifting up of some spiritual gifts—and the gifted people that exercise them—substantively different than the gift-glorifying error seen in 1 Corinthians 12–14?[12] Since the answer is "very little," those involved in such ministries must become aware that such an ongoing approach may produce rapid numerical growth, but it almost never fosters the spiritual maturity desperately needed in both recovery and discipleship over time.

Lingering Lesson III

Spiritual immaturity makes imbalanced, undiscerning responses. Now we turn to the way that maturity thinks and acts. There are two classic examples in 1 Corinthians that continue in 2 Corinthians.

The first example relates to the childlike (1 Cor. 3:1–2) tendency that the Corinthians had to form rival fan clubs (1:11–13; 3:3–9). What immaturity construes as jealous competition among chosen heroes, maturity sees as complementary ministry by fellow servants (1:13; 3:5–9).

The Corinthians, however, didn't learn much in the way of discernment from what happened. In 2 Corinthians 10–11 we find that many of the immature disciples in Corinth had been spellbound by Jewish false teachers. This time it wasn't just the jealous stupidity of fan clubs; it was the dangerous lack of discernment about the heretical nature of the teaching and lifestyle of those "false apostles" (11:13).

The second example has to do with the man having an affair with his stepmother, which Paul sternly rebukes in 1 Corinthians 5:1–5. His immature readers had apparently been arrogantly congratulating themselves about their open-mindedness in regard to the situation (v. 2). Paul, however, requires expulsion from the congregation (vv. 3–5)!

Some time later, after this man had truly repented, he sought to be restored to fellowship. Sadly, though, the same immature Corinthian disciples who had failed to discipline the man in the first place now refused to forgive and accept him back (2 Cor. 2:5–11). In other words, in one case they go to one undiscerning extreme, then, in the next related situation, they do a pendulum swing to the opposite extreme.

In this regard, we do well to hear and heed Paul's parting exhortations to his troublesome, immature readers in 1 Corinthians 16:13–14: "Be on the alert, stand firm in the faith, act like men, be strong. Let all that you do be done in love." This is not a frustrated demand to "Grow up!" but rather a balanced, mature tough love in action, seeking to help the beloved get beyond the rut of immaturity![13]

Lingering Lesson IV

Spiritual maturity understands that God's power works through weakness. The final lesson is seen in Paul's own experience in 2 Corinthians 12. To keep the apostle from immature self-exaltation, the Lord had given Paul a "thorn in the flesh" (i.e., some sort of painful bodily affliction; v. 7). This affliction had left the apostle very weak (v. 9), exactly the opposite of the "strong, natural leader" type so often idolized as spiritual giants by those who are spiritually immature.

It is the mature thing to be honest about our weaknesses (v. 10). It also is a spiritually mature realization that the Lord delights in working powerfully through weak vessels (vv. 9–10) to accomplish his ends, because he gets the glory. It is only when the disciple ceases to try to play from natural strength and gives his or her weaknesses (and strengths) over to the Lord that real progress in recovery or discipleship toward spiritual maturity can take place.[14]

8

Recovering the New Self

Ephesians and Colossians

In a recent article in *Christianity Today*, Andres Tapia discussed the unique problems and challenges the baby buster[1] generation presents to the contemporary evangelical church. He argues quite persuasively throughout the article that the church is going to have to radically transform its approach to ministry in order to reach this post-Christian generation.

Quoting from several authorities, Tapia gives a brief background on Generation X (baby busters) and also delineates some of its major characteristics:

> If, indeed, the church must change its approach to reach the Xers, it must first understand the essence of the brief but complex history of the 38 million individuals who make up Generation X.
>
> They are the children of divorce, with 50 percent coming from broken homes; and they are the children of two-job families, where parents often were not around.

In their book *13th Gen* (for the thirteenth generation to grow up under the U.S. flag), Neil Howe and Bill Strauss predict that given their dysfunctional family background, Xers will be incarcerated and executed at a higher rate than any previous generation in U.S. history. According to their statistics, every day 13 youth commit suicide, 16 are murdered, 1,000 become mothers, 100,000 bring guns to school, 500 begin using drugs, 1,000 begin drinking alcohol, 3,500 are assaulted, 630 are robbed, and 80 are raped.

These sobering realities have produced a generation pessimistic about its own chances. Barna says baby busters "are the most ignored, misunderstood, and disheartened generation our country has seen in a long time." Richard Peace, professor of evangelism at Fuller Theological Seminary, calls this a "clinically depressed generation."[2]

Tapia adds further that Generation X is looking for answers from the church and is basically in search of five things: authenticity, community, abandonment of dogmatism, a focus on the arts, and diversity.[3] Whether you are a baby buster or not, if you are struggling with recovery issues, you are probably longing for some of these very things.

We would readily agree that the evangelical church should transform some of its ministries in order to meet the needs of Christians (that is, baby boomers, baby busters, and beyond!) who are in recovery. The church, according to the biblical pattern (see Eph. 4:1–16; Col. 3:12–17), should naturally be a place of openness, honesty, and community.

We are reluctant, however, to fully endorse all of Tapia's solutions for the recovery-related problems facing this generation and the church. For instance, we do not believe the answer is to radically contextualize Jesus so as to make him more suitable to this culture. Contextualization can be dangerous in that we run the risk of presenting a Jesus who is completely foreign to the Jesus of the Gospels.

Besides, Jesus is not the one in need of transformation. *We* are the ones who need to change. Jesus has made our transformation possible by sacrificing himself. It is in his death and resurrection that our true self is rediscovered. God is in the process of re-creating us in the image of his Son.

In Ephesians and Colossians, Paul speaks of this re-creation as the "new self" (Eph. 4:24; Col. 3:10). It is in the new self that we find our true identity and purpose. The authenticity and community that the baby busters (and everyone else) desire is only achieved in putting off the old self and living through the new self (Eph. 4:22–24).

From a discipleship and recovery standpoint, the apostle Paul's discourses in Ephesians and Colossians concerning the headship of Christ, the new self, and unity is highly relevant. Paul provides steadfast answers to a contemporary generation in need of discipleship and recovery and presents to us in context the Jesus of the Gospels.

Discipleship and Recovery Themes in Ephesians and Colossians

The similarities between Ephesians and Colossians have been widely recognized by evangelical biblical scholars.[4] Many of the common themes are pertinent to both discipleship and recovery. The most obvious similarities are found in the themes mentioned above: the headship of Christ, the new self, and unity.

We will explore these topics and how they specifically relate to discipleship and recovery throughout the rest of this chapter. However, for now we want to make mention of other commonalities that are not so obvious but are relevant to our current discussion. These have to do with Paul's situation at the time he penned the letters and with the circumstances surrounding the churches at Ephesus and Colossae.

It is generally held that Paul wrote Ephesians and Colossians during his first imprisonment at Rome (Acts 28:30–31).[5] Paul was in an extremely precarious situation. His life lay in the hands of the Roman government, and he had very little idea when he would finally face Caesar. So, with his future yet uncertain, Paul turned his heart to other more important matters.

We must remember that, while Paul was an apostle, he was still a growing disciple. He was the first to attest that he had not yet arrived to a state of Christlike perfection (Phil. 3:12). He was in the process of learning and growing just like those to whom he ministered. He was, however, a *mature* disciple, and this is seen most clearly in the content of his letters to the Ephesians and Colossians.

The apostle could have been bitter about his circumstances and indulged in self-pity. Instead, he was caught up with concern for those entrusted to him. His compassion and concern flowed through his pen as he expounded on the doctrine of Christ, the new self, and unity. He gave those churches (and us) what they needed to continue on the path to discipleship.

Considering Paul's situation, recovery issues could have consumed him, but it is clear that he chose to put into practice the very things he wrote to the Ephesians and Colossians. He spoke from authority not only as one inspired by the Holy Spirit, but also as one who practiced what he preached. In this regard, he is an example to all disciples who struggle with recovery issues.

The circumstances facing the churches at Ephesus and Colossae were quite different. For example, the church at Colossae was being threatened by heretical teachings. Paul was determined to expose these false doctrines, so his letter to the Colossian church is polemic and purposeful in nature.[6]

The churches at Ephesus and the surrounding Asian province were not dealing with such controversies.[7] They were generally at peace. Hence, Paul's approach is much more relaxed and contemplative. The Ephesian letter is meditative in nature and theologically profound. The apostle expanded on many of the doctrines the Colossian letter contains only in capsule form.

Considering the different situations facing the Ephesian and Colossian churches, it makes sense that Paul's style and approach would be different in each letter. What is interesting and relevant to our discussion, however, is that Paul's basic message to each church is strikingly similar.

The point seems to be clear that, no matter what situation we are facing, the message of Ephesians and Colossians can provide sufficient answers. Whether we are being inundated by the lies of people who wish to take advantage of us or whether we are simply desiring the deeper things of God, the truths contained in these letters can help us.

Ephesians and Colossians teach us that both discipleship and recovery involve the consistent application of spiritual truths in our lives. The discipleship and recovery we seek is accomplished only through the daily living out of these crucial spiritual realities.

The Headship of Christ

In Ephesians 1:10, Christ is pictured as the head over all things in heaven and earth. The entire universe will be brought together under his headship. Wood explains:

> The verb *anakephalaioō* ("to bring together") means to sum up together again. . . . It is derived not from *kephalē* ("a head") but from *kephalaion* ("a summary, or sum total"). When a column of figures was added up, the total was placed at the top. At the end of the age everything will be seen to add up to Christ. This recognition of his preeminence will ensure that the original harmony of the universe is restored. . . . The mission of Christ extends beyond the human race and assumes cosmic dimensions.[8]

With this incredible revelation of Christ's all-encompassing authority in view, the apostle Paul sets the stage to show Christ's role as head over the church: "And God placed all things under his feet and appointed him to be head over everything for the church, which is his body, the fullness of him who fills everything in every way" (Eph. 1:22–23 NIV).

Foulkes eloquently points out that "there is given to the Church, and for the Church's benefit, a head who is also head over all things. The Church has authority and power to overcome all opposition because her leader and head is Lord of all."[9]

This fact is strikingly pertinent to both discipleship and recovery. Christ holds all power and authority in the universe (Eph. 1:19–21). Because we are members of his body and vitally connected to him, there is no obstacle big enough to permanently hinder us on the road to discipleship and recovery.

This idea of Christ's supremacy is expressed even more strongly in the Book of Colossians:

> For by him all things were created: things in heaven and on earth, visible and invisible, whether thrones or powers or rulers or author-

ities; all things were created by him and for him. He is before all things, and in him all things hold together. And he is the head of the body, the church; he is the beginning and the firstborn from among the dead, so that in everything he might have the supremacy.

Colossians 1:16–19 NIV

When applied to the discipleship and recovery process, the truth of Christ's headship and authority can bring real comfort and power. In Ephesians 4:15 Paul tells us that we are to "grow up into him who is the Head" (NIV). Wood gives extraordinary insight into the context of these verses: "Paul contrasts the deception of heresy with the integrity of the gospel. The church cannot allow falsehood to go uncorrected, yet the truth must always be vindicated in the accents of love. . . . This fundamental concern for the truth is the secret of maturity in the church."[10]

As we grow up into him who is the head, our maturity must express itself in love and support of one another. This kind of spiritual maturity can only be fully expressed through the new self.

The New Self

For those who come from an abusive background or have been involved in unhealthy relationships, anger, bitterness, and resentment are usually a big problem. In a real sense, these attitudes are natural reactions to such experiences. As Christians, though, these people have a hard time coping with these undesirable feelings.

They long to let go of these feelings because of the negative impact they have on every aspect of their lives. An even deeper dilemma comes into play when these hurting Christians read Bible verses such as the following from Ephesians and Colossians:

Get rid of all bitterness, rage and anger, brawling and slander, along with every form of malice. Be kind and compassionate to one another, forgiving each other, just as in Christ God forgave you.

Ephesians 4:31–32 NIV

> But now you must rid yourselves of all such things as these: anger, rage, malice, slander, and filthy language from your lips. . . . Therefore, as God's chosen people, holy and dearly loved, clothe yourselves with compassion, kindness, humility, gentleness and patience. Bear with each other and forgive whatever grievances you may have against one another.
>
> Colossians 3:8, 12–13 NIV

A natural question arises from the minds of those who read these penetrating passages: How do I "rid" and "forgive"? All disciples of Christ have a deep desire to obey God's Word and do what is right, but for recovering disciples who struggle intensely with negative emotions, these commands may seem almost impossible.

However, a more intimate understanding of the immediate context of these passages may bring some comfort and relief and alleviate a lot of guilt and confusion. Yes, these imperatives apply to *all* disciples across the board, and it must be our goal to obey them. But the commands must be understood and obeyed in light of the overall context of the passage.

The New Testament writers describe the new life in Christ in various ways.[11] In Colossians and Ephesians, the apostle Paul describes it as putting off the old self and putting on the new self. Guthrie gives some insight into Paul's usage of these terms:

> The resurrection experience understood in a corporate sense comes over clearly in Colossians 3:1ff. In this passage the dying results in life being hidden with Christ in God, that is to say that life gains a new centre, which although less manifest than the old is nevertheless more real. It means seeking higher things and thinking in higher modes of thought. The resurrection involves a complete transformation of the way of life. The old life has to be resolutely put to death, a fate which it deserves, and conversely the new life has to be embraced.[12]

The passages quoted above (Eph. 4:31–32; Col. 3:8, 12–13) must be understood in the context of putting to death the old self and putting on the new self (Eph. 4:22–23; Col. 3:9). What Paul does in Ephesians and Colossians is to boldly set forth the characteristics of the old and the new self so there is no confusion as to what behavior belongs to which.

The apostle then exhorts the churches to live in accordance with the new self simply because that is who they really are. As Guthrie points out, the death and resurrection of Jesus made the new self a living reality and gave life a whole "new centre." In other words, the new self manifests Christlike character, is a life centered in him, and is a life empowered by him.

Yet the questions still arise: How is this putting on and putting off accomplished? It is something we do, or is it done for us by Christ? Is it a onetime thing, or is it a process? Guthrie provides us with some answers:

> Paul gives a list of vices which the Christians are exhorted to put to death. The list includes sins of the mind like impurity, evil desire and covetousness. To put these to death means again a radical approach to one's mental state. It involves no less than a moral revolution. The old nature with its practices must be resolutely put away. But is Paul suggesting that each person must put off the old nature before he can hope to put on the new? This would impose an intolerable burden on the individual and would smack too much of works to be a plausible understanding of Paul's thought. The only reasonable interpretation is to suppose that "putting off" and "putting on" are opposing sides of one action. It is only when the new nature is embraced that the old nature can be put to death. The apostle gives no indication that this putting off is a once-for-all operation except in an ideal sense. . . . It is rather a process, in short, the process of sanctification.[13]

It is crucial to both discipleship and recovery that we continue in the process of sanctification. Embracing and cherishing the new self assures us that we are growing and progressing on that path.

Remember, our goal as Christ's disciples is not happiness but holiness! The pursuit of holiness will have as natural by-products both happiness and healthy relationships.

A Community in Unity

As we pointed out at the beginning of this chapter, the baby busters are a generation searching for identity, purpose, authenticity, and community. As we have seen, the apostle Paul, in his letters to the Ephesians and Colossians, offers some solutions to these challenges.

Christ, who is the head over every power and authority, gives his people a new identity (the new self) and purpose. He empowers the new self to exude Christ's character. With all of this, he has created us to be a community of people able to live together in unity. The universal church is the firstfruits of all things that will be brought together under his headship.

A major theme in the Book of Ephesians is unity, especially between Jew and Gentile. For our purposes, let us briefly examine this theme and how it fits into the book's overall argument. In a broad sense, the epistle can be divided into two sections: the cause (chaps. 1–3) and the effect (chaps. 4–6).

The church is divinely ordained, chosen, blessed, and empowered from the heavenly realms by Christ (chap. 1). Jew and Gentile have been brought together in the church and made one in Christ (chaps. 2–3). As a result, all believers (especially Jew and Gentile) must be unified in spirit, heart, and mind (chap. 4). In addition, it is imperative that believers conduct themselves in all their relationships in complete holiness in accordance with their heavenly calling (chaps. 5–6).

Paul begins this profound epistle by setting forth God's foreordained plan of salvation. God's plan to redeem the elect was in his mind long before the creation of the world. The adoption of believers as his children through Jesus Christ was done in accordance with his pleasure and will. This is an amazing thought in light of the fact that we had nothing to offer him but our sin and rebellion.

The apostle makes it clear from the beginning that God's ultimate purpose in the plan of salvation was "to bring all things in heaven and earth together under one head, even Christ" (Eph. 1:10 NIV). The church as a spiritual unity is the blessed recipient of the riches of God's grace by which the mystery of his will was made known.

Paul also ends his letter on a spiritual note. His focus, however, is not on the glories and riches of the heavenly realm but on the wiles of the devil, who wrecks havoc in that realm. The "spiritual battle" section of this letter (Eph. 6:10–24) is one of the most popular and well-known in all of Scripture, but the battle is not always understood properly. In order to get a clear picture of what Paul is talking about, we must consider the broad and, especially, the immediate context surrounding this critical passage.

The apostle has taken us full circle. He began the letter with an emphasis on Christ in the heavenly realm and ended it with a discussion of the enemy who dwells in the same heavenly realm. This is in no way out of place for this practical, down-to-earth section of the letter (chaps. 4–6).

In fact, Paul has been progressively building his readers to the point of understanding the harmony between the spiritual and the practical. He moved from the spiritual realm to the physical, human implications of that realm in chapters 1–3, then from the earthly domain to the spiritual implications of that domain in chapters 4–6.

After Paul led us through the practical meaning of the truths revealed in the opening chapters (1–3), he showed that unity, maturity, and Christlikeness must characterize the corporate church and all human relationships (4:1–6:9). This is the immediate context of the spiritual battle section (6:10–24).

The devil's game plan, then, is to break up the key human relationships Paul had just been talking about in Ephesians 5:22–6:9. Thus, we must understand the unseen battle in this context. Satan is the enemy of all harmony and unity.

Therefore, we must be on guard against any disruption of community. One of Satan's prime tactics is to get us to resurrect the old self (chaps. 4–5) and embrace those negative emotions associated with it. These naturally lead to disharmony.

The point Paul is making in the placement of the spiritual battle section is that godly character (the new self) will be a crucial part of our defense against the spiritual enemy of unity and community. Satan's attack is subtle and deadly, so we must always be ready with the full armor of godly character and God-given resources.

The apostle has made it clear throughout the Ephesian letter that the Christian calling and experience is not merely earthly. The church clearly exists in two realms. Therefore, we must be armed with the knowledge of the power and authority of Christ, be clothed with the new self, and be persistent in pursuing unity. These things are absolutely essential for the discipleship and recovery process to proceed on as they should.

9

Twin Case Studies in Intervention

Philemon and Philippians

It is common to hear someone refer to "making a mountain out of a molehill." By that it is usually meant a problem is being escalated way out of proportion to its original (or actual) significance.

Come to think of it, though, I have never heard anyone speak of "making a molehill out of a mountain." This would, of course, imply scaling down a big problem or dispute to a much smaller level, at which resolution and/or reconciliation is workable.

The difficulty is that an escalated "mountain" often requires outside intervention before it can begin to be deflated to "molehill" size. That is very often the case when various kinds of recovery issues have escalated out of control. A person, couple, or family in such circumstances simply cannot get a handle on the "molehill become a mountain" on their own and are headed for disaster. They desperately need help from he or she is who knows what they are doing, and they need it *now!*[1]

From a general standpoint, virtually every letter in the New Testament is attempting to "make a molehill out of a mountain." Each Epistle attempts to deal with problems among the disciples being addressed. Thus, they each represent a sort of Christian intervention.

Side-by-Side Scriptural Searchlights on Intervention

Two of the letters that reflect the most direct kind of intervention were written from the same location and circumstances in a surprisingly similar format (and, likely, within months or even weeks of each other, with Philemon only slightly earlier). Strangely, for all their similarities, the "twin epistles" of Philemon and Philippians are seldom considered side by side.[2]

Since it is not unheard of to yoke the two letters together,[3] however, we will pursue what they have to say about intervention individually and together. The amazing extent of the parallels between Philemon and Philippians is displayed in table 9.1.

Table 9.1
Two Strikingly Similar Letters from Paul

Philemon*	Parallel Aspects	Philippians**
Paul and Timothy	Stated authors (intervenors)	Paul and Timothy
Paul's jail cell	Place of writing	Paul's jail cell
A.D. 61 or 62	Date of writing	A.D. 61 or 62
Philemon	Focal person(s) requiring intervention	Euodia and Syntyche
Fellow worker	Description of focal person(s)	Fellow workers
Beloved; partner	Closeness to Paul	Beloved; partners
Onesimus	Person(s) sent to work on reconciliation	Epaphroditus (and Timothy)
Onesimus served Paul in jail	Previous role	Epaphroditus served Paul in jail

Philemon*	Parallel Aspects	Philippians**
Accept Onesimus as a brother; as me	Paul's appeal	Accept Timothy as "my son" and a model
To visit Philemon	Paul's plans	To visit Philippi
Reader's prayers	Basis for plans	Readers' prayers
Recognize new status in Christ	Solution	Swallow pride, selfishness
Onesimus	Beneficiary	Philippian church

*Helpful, though slightly differing, evangelical discussions of background issues related to Philemon can be found in Howard F. Vos, "Philemon," in *Evangelical Commentary on the Bible*, ed. Walter A. Elwell (Grand Rapids: Baker, 1989), 1119; and D. A. Carson, Douglas J. Moo, and Leon Morris, *An Introduction to the New Testament* (Grand Rapids: Zondervan, 1992), 387–89.
**Conservative discussions of the background of Philippians can be found in A. Boyd Luter, "Philippians," in *Evangelical Commentary*, ed. Elwell, 1034–37; and Carson, Moo, and Morris, *Introduction to the New Testament*, 317–22.

Such a table is an excellent way to quickly survey the similar background, themes, and objectives of these two epistles. Still, it does not convey the full range of similarity.

Kindred Thought Cast in the Same Mold

Strikingly, both Philemon and Philippians are notably alike in their literary structure. Though Philippians is considerably longer, both are arranged in inverted parallel form (or chiasm), an approach that emphasizes by facing off themes in the first and second halves of the structure.[4]

There was a time when it was thought that chiastic structuring was an almost entirely Semitic literary approach.[5] However, in the past decades, more and more studies have emerged (and are now coming out in volume) that demonstrate the widespread presence of such structural inversion even in New Testament books written to churches with relatively little Jewish makeup or background.[6] That description would certainly seem to characterize Philemon and Philippians.[7]

The following two outlines provide an overview survey of the flow and relationships of thought in Philemon, then Philippians. As was noted in table 9.1, there are notable, specific differences between the letters, given the different occasions for which they were written. Yet, the similarities in background, themes, and, as seen below, literary structure are more prevalent.

An Initially "Private" Intervention: Philemon

A. Opening greetings between fellow workers (vv. 1–3)
  B. Prayerful commendation of Philemon, a partner and brother (vv. 4–7)
    C. Personal intervention for Onesimus, a slave and brother (vv. 8–16)
  B[1]. Personal accountability as a partner and brother, expecting prayer (vv. 17–22)
A[1]. Closing greetings from fellow workers (vv. 23–25)[8]

Obviously, the modest length of Paul's Epistle to Philemon (i.e., one chapter of twenty-five verses) gives the appearance that it is little more than a short, intensely personal note from the apostle to his friend, Philemon. Thus, the reader might tend to think that since Philippians is considerably longer (four chapters), it would be more carefully crafted structurally than Philemon.

Interestingly, though, Philippians has often faced much the same rap as Philemon. It has also been viewed as a short, personal letter with little or no discernible structure.[9] The following outline attempts to dispel that kind of shortsighted misconception.

A Sensitively "Public" Intervention: Philippians[10]

A. Opening greetings: Previewing "partnership in the gospel" theme and emphasizing humble leadership (1:1–2)
  B. Prologue: Partnership in the gospel theme introduced, with prayerful gratitude (1:3–11)
    C. Comfort/Example: Paul's safety and right thinking in the midst of a difficult, "guarded" situation (1:12–26)

    D. Challenge: Stand fast and be united, fulfilling Paul's joy as a partner (1:27–2:4)

        E. Example/Action: Christ's example of humility and suffering before glory, then related behavioral instructions (2:5–16)

        F.   Midpoint: Caring models of gospel partnership, two of which are sent to help (2:17–3:1a)

      E^1. Example/Action: Paul's example of humbling and identification with Christ's suffering before the "upward call," then instructions (3:1b–21)

    D^1. Challenge: Stand fast and accentuate existing joy by the reconciliation of two gospel partners (4:1–5)

  C^1. Comfort/Example: The Philippians had "guarded" peace of mind and right thinking in the midst of an anxious situation (4:6–9)

 B^1. Epilogue: Partnership from the past renewed and remembered, with expressed gratitude (4:10–20)

A^1. Closing greetings: Reviewing partnership in the gospel theme, emphasizing unity of the saints (4:21–23)[11]

We have now gotten a general sense of how Paul laid out Philemon and Philippians as, so to speak, structural twins to speak to the problems requiring intervention in each setting. It remains to explore the exact nature of each situation, how the apostle handled things, and the apparent goals he sought to achieve in each case, which will provide the bottom-line implications for recovery and discipleship. That will be done by a more up-close-and-personal, side by side comparison.

The Problems in Which Paul Intervened

In regard to the circumstances that prompted Paul to write both Philemon and Philippians, significant relationships involving relatively mature disciples had seriously deteriorated. In both cases, the resulting distance had to be bridged and healed. It is not at all certain, though, that these long-standing disciples were ready, willing, and able to face up to the problems at hand.

As seen in table 9.1, Philemon, Euodia, and Syntyche were all described as "beloved" and "fellow worker(s)" (Philem. 1; Phil. 4:2–3). Since *fellow worker* (Greek *sunergos*) is a term that implies commitment to a shared mission, it certainly implies a significant degree of, so to speak, playing-on-the-same-team discipleship (i.e., with Paul, for Christ). It also is a term that the apostle delighted to use but did not take lightly.[12] For example, in Philemon the only other use of "fellow worker(s)" is in verse 24, referring to the handful of ministry lieutenants who had stood by Paul through his imprisonment (v. 13). In Philippians, the elements of commitment and relationship are even more obvious, since the lone additional usage refers to Epaphroditus (Phil. 2:25). After all, Epaphroditus courageously served both the Philippian church and the apostle and almost lost his life in the process (vv. 25–30).

Despite their undoubted commitment to the Lord (and Paul) and their level of maturity as disciples, however, there was no apparent willingness on the parts of Philemon or Euodia and Syntyche to resolve the mountainlike conflicts they were mired in. From all appearances, their attitudes were very close to the classic "I have been wronged, and I have every right to be angry and bitter!"

Philemon's slave, Onesimus, had fled, eventually to Rome (Philem. 10–12). That had deprived Philemon not only of a needed worker but also a valuable piece of property.[13] He was apparently very upset at the loss, and it was well within his legal rights to punish Onesimus harshly—if and when he got him back![14] In the meantime, though, Onesimus had become a Christian in Rome through Paul (vv. 10–11). Yet Philemon was still viewing Onesimus as lost or stolen property.

At roughly the same time in Philippi, a dispute of some sort[15] had erupted between Euodia and Syntyche (Phil. 4:2–3). Though "anger" and "bitterness" are too often present in the church (Eph. 4:31), this situation escalated to the point of significantly affecting the wider congregation and infringing on Paul's joy toward them (Phil. 2:2–4).[16] That point was underlined by the parallel "challenge" sections in the outline of Philippians (see D and D1).

With the church in Philippi facing mounting *external* dangers (1:28–30; 3:2–4), it was past time for them to get their *internal* house in order! But that could not be done in any comprehensive sense as long as Euodia and Syntyche, two apparently higher-profile disciples locally in the cause of the spread of the gospel, refused to budge an inch to defuse their dispute.

These were the twin relational San Andreas faults in which the apostle determined he must intervene, even if it was from his jail cell! But note that he chose to do so *before* they hit bottom,[17] before they had an earthquakelike shattering impact on these individuals (and churches) he cared so much about (Phil. 1:3–11, esp. vv. 7–8; Col. 1:3–8; Philem. 4–7).

The Means and Ends of Paul's Interventions

Significantly, in both cases Paul began and framed his intervention in positive tones. He complimented them as "partner" disciples (Phil. 1:5; Philem. 6, 17) and appealed to them in the context of being "beloved" spiritual family members (Phil. 4:1; Philem. 1, 7, 20).

Then, before he made his specific appeals (Phil. 4:2–3; Philem. 10–20), the apostle set up the confrontations in general terms. With Philemon it took the form of refusing to wield his authority as an apostle but rather speaking out of the context of his own limitations (Philem. 8–9). In other words, Paul refused to bulldoze Philemon or treat him like a child, but rather he treated him as another respected adult disciple of Christ!

With Euodia and Syntyche the stage was set by a discrete general appeal to the entire Philippian church to "make my joy complete by being of the same mind" (Phil. 2:2) and facing up to prideful self-interest (vv. 3–4). With unity being such a key mark of a maturing church body (Eph. 4:13),[18] all the disciples in the Philippian church needed to hear this admonition. However, with the mushrooming cold war between Euodia and Syntyche likely threatening to tear apart the very fabric of the church's unity, everyone was put on alert that Paul was seeking to intervene in a lovingly sensitive, but firm, manner.

Then in Philippians 4:2–3 the apostle's tough love moved into face-to-face position! Refusing to be drawn into taking sides, Paul carefully (individually) exhorted both women (v. 2).[19] He also appealed to someone only referred to as "true comrade" (v. 3) to help with the intervention as an on-the-scene accountability figure.

So what did Paul want to see accomplished? In both cases, forgiving reconciliation. That way Onesimus could return to Philemon, now as a spiritual brother, not just a slave (Philem. 14–17). And Euodia and Syntyche could be joyfully reunited as veteran, teammate disciples, rebuilding the fractured unity of that church (Phil. 2:2–4; 4:2–3).

So What Difference Did It Make?

Was the calculated risk of these twin interventions successful? There is no way of knowing absolutely, since there is no later scriptural mention of any of these disciples. Yet it seems likely that these New Testament case studies are presented with the decided implication that all involved did face their problems, forgive, and reconstruct much healthier relationships.[20]

The bottom-line principles here relate to both recovery and discipleship:

1. Even fairly mature disciples can too easily trap themselves in situations that require intervention.
2. Loving Christian intervention should not wait for circumstances to escalate to the point where the disciples involved hit bottom.
3. The intervention should be done discretely and sensitively, but firmly.
4. The goal is forgiving reconciliation and restoration.

That's the apostle Paul's sage, inspired (2 Tim. 3:16) advice on deflating emotional/relational mountains into molehills!

10

Be Ready for Recovery

1–2 Thessalonians

Imagine yourself in this scenario: You're walking along a road one day when you are met by someone who tells you about a man in a distant land who loved you so much that he died for you. You are also told that this same man rose from the dead and ascended into heaven with a promise to return one day and take those who believe in him back to his heavenly home.

Initially, you think the story sounds very far-fetched, if not crazy. But there is something about the messenger that holds your attention. His words are always gracious and encouraging, and he seems to genuinely love and care for everyone who comes to hear him.

Slowly, his teachings begin to make sense to you. His actions move you and finally prove to you the truthfulness of his message. You believe, and your life is changed. You continue to bask in this man's love, growing in the grace and knowledge of the God he introduced to you.

Then suddenly it happens! The trials and persecutions he warned you about relentlessly fall upon you. The good news this messenger preached has put your community in an uproar, and you receive the brunt of their anger. Frantically, you call upon this man you've grown to trust, but he's nowhere to be found. You search for him but come up empty.

The townspeople inform you that he has left. "He deserted you in your time of trouble," they say. Your people continue to ruthlessly mock and ridicule you for having believed such a charlatan. They jeer you, "He was a liar and a cheat from the beginning and cared nothing for you! Now you alone must face the consequences for having been so gullible." But you really thought for sure that he and his God were sincere.

The Perils of Persecution

Maybe it's not hard for you to imagine yourself in the above situation because you've had a similar experience. If so, you will be able to more deeply understand the first century Thessalonian believers and their relationship to the apostle Paul, for the story depicts in broad brush strokes what happened to them. Even if you cannot relate to their experience, though, there is much to be learned from the letters Paul wrote to the Thessalonians.

Paul, along with his companions, Silas and Timothy, visited Thessalonica on his second missionary journey (Acts 15:36–40; 17:1). He was there for at least three weeks (three Sabbaths) reasoning with the Jews and God-fearing Greeks in their synagogue, trying to convince them that Jesus was the Christ (17:2–3). However, based on the apparent depth of relationship between Paul and the Thessalonians (1 Thess. 2:7–12), there is a good possibility that he was there longer than just three weeks.[1]

Some of the Jews and many of the Gentiles believed Paul's message and became disciples of Jesus (Acts 17:4). This response stirred up the Jews and made them jealous. So they gathered up some of the worst characters they could find in the marketplace and started a riot in the city. The angry mob stormed the house of a man by the name of Jason in search of Paul and his friends (17:5).

When they could not find Paul, they dragged Jason out of his house and brought him before the officials, accusing him of housing Paul and defying Caesar by proclaiming Jesus as king (17:6–7). The unbelievers apparently interpreted Paul's message about Jesus to mean a possible threat to Caesar and his kingdom. This was a serious charge, and the city officials took it as such, for they were all thrown into turmoil. They made Jason post bond for Paul and his companions as if they were members of his own household (17:8–9).[2]

Because of the intensity of the situation, some of the believers, possibly Jason and his friends, decided to send Paul and Silas on to Berea (17:10), located fifty-five miles southwest of Thessalonica.[3] However, the trials and persecution did not end with Paul's departure. The believers who were left behind, those who were a faithful witness to Jesus Christ, were greatly persecuted by their community (see 1 Thess. 2:14; 3:2–3; 2 Thess. 1:4–5).

So, at a time when these new converts needed Paul the most, he was nowhere to be found! The one they had rapidly grown to trust seemed, for all practical purposes, to have deserted them. His comfort and encouragement were desperately needed to calm their fears, but he was gone. Paul, however, was very much aware of their unbearable situation and wrote to assure them that he did not desert them. He was not the swindler and deceiver his enemies were making him out to be (1 Thess. 2:1–12).

On the contrary, Paul sincerely loved them, cared about their situation, and earnestly made every effort to see them (2:17–18). Satan may have been able to block him from physically coming to the Thessalonians, but he could not hinder Paul's love or concern for them. In his place, Paul sent Timothy to visit these new believers and penned his first letter to them in order to assure them of his good intentions.

This message of love and concern that God had spoken through Paul to the Thessalonian believers is strongly applicable to disciples in recovery today. Sometimes it may seem as though God has left us alone to face the trials and persecutions of life. It may seem he has turned a deaf ear to our cries for deliverance, but 1–2 Thessalonians assure us that this is simply not the case.

The apostle Paul was a true messenger sent by God (1 Thess. 2:3–6, 13). Therefore, we can completely trust what Paul has taught about God. He assures us that God is aware of and deeply concerned for his persecuted saints (1 Thess. 1:4; 2 Thess. 1:4–5; 2:13; 3:5). God has promised ultimate deliverance for those who have suffered for his name. This truth also extends to his people who are suffering from past wounds. Though their afflictions may not be a direct result of their witness for Christ, God still cares about their pain and hears their cries for mercy.

In these epistles, Paul encourages the persecuted Thessalonian believers with the hope of the second coming of Christ and a bright, pain-free future (1 Thess. 1:10; 2:19; 3:13; 4:13–18; 5:23; 2 Thess. 1:7–10; 2:8). He reminds them that those who are persecuting them will receive their just punishment when Christ returns. These truths can serve to encourage recovering believers not to take revenge on their persecutors but to wait upon the Lord, who will rescue them and give them eternal hope for the future.

Actively Waiting

In some evangelical circles, the word *rescue* has become much more associated with codependency than with the second coming of Christ. The problem of the codependent rescuing an addicted loved one from his or her drug of choice has overshadowed the glorious truth that Christ will return and rescue us from the coming wrath (1 Thess. 1:10).

Christ's return is the kind of rescue we can all eagerly anticipate as his disciples, and it is a good and healthy rescue! Christ has delivered us from God's wrath against sin, and, at his return, we will experience complete relief from all trials and persecutions. These truths give us hope in the present and promise for the future. The doctrine of the second coming should motivate us to pursue discipleship and recovery. As the apostle Paul warns us, we must not be idle; we must be actively waiting for his return! (See 1 Thess. 4:1, 11–12; 5:6, 14; 2 Thess. 3:6–15).

Warren Wiersbe eloquently points out that "Paul did not look on this doctrine [of the second coming] as a theory to be discussed, but as a truth to be lived. These letters encourage us to live 'in the future tense' since Jesus could appear at any time. We are to practice the promise of His return in our manner of life."[4]

Wiersbe also gives a brief but helpful thematic outline of 1 Thessalonians, showing how the doctrine of the second coming relates practically to many aspects of Christian living:

1:10	salvation and assurance
2:19–20	soul-winning and service
3:11–13	stability in Christian living
4:13–18	strength for sorrow
5:23–24	sanctification of life

One of Paul's primary purposes for writing 1–2 Thessalonians was to motivate us into action as disciples of Christ. The apostle stresses in the verses in the above outline that the future hope of Christ's return should impact our behavior in the here and now. These passages also serve to encourage us in the recovery process, in which we are actively, not passively, involved.

The ingredient needed for both discipleship and recovery to progress in a healthy and productive manner is hope. The promise of the second coming of Christ offers this hope in abundance. When true biblical hope is applied to our lives on a daily basis, it can give us a whole new perspective on the various trials and sufferings we constantly face.

The way we use the word *hope* in our day can rob it of its rich biblical meaning. For instance, "I hope I get the job," or "I hope I find the right person to marry someday" are common statements in which *hope* is used to express our desire for something to happen. In this usage there is always a considerable element of uncertainty because things might not turn out the way we want them to. There is always the real possibility that our desires may not come to pass.

This is not true of *hope* in the biblical context, especially as it is used for the second coming. This biblical hope is actually a *guarantee* of what is to come. There is no way that it will not come to pass! Vine describes the usage of the word in the context of Christ's return in this way:

[Hope] (*elpis*), in the N.T., [is defined as] favourable and confident expectation. . . . Hope is a factor in salvation, Rom. 8:24; it finds

its expression in endurance under trial, which is the effect of waiting for the Coming of Christ, 1 Thess. 1:3. . . . It is a purifying power,
"every one that hath this hope set on Him purifieth himself, even
as He is pure," 1 John 3:3.[5]

Salvation, service, stability, strength, and sanctification work
together in us to produce hope, which is inspired by the *sure* coming of our Lord Jesus Christ. Therefore, we are to remain steadfast
in the faith and live in the light of this future reality.

To live consistently "in the future tense," as Wiersbe puts it,
presents a real problem for some believers, especially for those in
recovery. The pain and trials they are enduring in the present are
so intense that they totally obscure their hope for the future. They
wonder why God does not deliver them *today*. They wonder if he
has completely forgotten them. Hence, their hope gets lost in a
sea of despair.

In a sense, this is what the Thessalonian believers began to experience, which produced the need for Paul to write 2 Thessalonians.
There was great confusion among some of the believers concerning the day of the Lord (2 Thess. 2:1–2). Some people had apparently spread rumors in the church that the day of the Lord had
already come and that they were somehow left behind.

The ever-increasing trials and persecutions these young converts were enduring seemed to confirm what they were being
told. In light of this, it is easy to understand their fear and despair.
They thought God had abandoned them in their time of greatest need (just like they thought Paul did after he first preached
the gospel to them).

Paul wrote 2 Thessalonians to restore hope to the believers by
informing them that God was keenly aware of their trials and
promised complete relief at the return of his Son (2 Thess. 1:6–7).
The Lord had not abandoned them. Paul warned them in his
first letter that they would be persecuted (1 Thess. 3:3–4), but
their sufferings would produce the perseverance needed to complete their faith. Therefore, he encouraged them not to be idle
but to continue as faithful witnesses of the Lord Jesus Christ
(2 Thess. 3:6–14).

We do not know if the Thessalonian believers ever experienced any earthly relief from their suffering. We do know for sure that none of them saw the coming of the Lord. But, because of 1–2 Thessalonians, we know that Paul was extending hope to them through the knowledge that Christ would return to claim them and judge their persecutors and that this hope was to be expressed in their daily lives through holy behavior.

These are the enduring and timeless principles contained in 1–2 Thessalonians. They are meant to strengthen and instruct disciples in every generation. They can also be a great source of encouragement to those who are in recovery. It is not our place to take revenge on our past or present persecutors. "For after all it is only just for *God* to repay with affliction those who afflict you" (2 Thess. 1:6; italics mine).

Nevertheless, we can and must pray, like Paul, that "we may be delivered from perverse and evil men; for not all have faith" (2 Thess. 3:2). The sad and difficult aspect of doing this is that we may be praying for deliverance from our own family members! The consolation, however, is that we can also pray that the Lord would free them from their vicious cycle of abuse and grant them the gift of salvation.

As we are waiting for God's Son, we should be actively working on discipleship and recovery. Idleness is the devil's playground and can wreck havoc in both of these crucial areas. Satan would like nothing more than for those who bear Christ's name to be caught in a web of sin that ruins their witness. It is vital that we actively pursue holiness and do no wrong to others. That way we will not be caught off guard at his coming; instead, we will be ready for the ultimate recovery, fully alert and self-controlled (1 Thess. 5:6).

Scriptural Truth with True Relationship

"Rejoice always; pray without ceasing; in everything give thanks; for this is God's will for you in Christ Jesus" (1 Thess. 5:16–18). If you have been a Christian for a while, you have probably had these verses quoted to you by well-meaning believers during a time of personal crisis.[6] These passages are frequently coupled with other spiritual statements that echo biblical truth:

"It's God's will for you to go through this."
"God is in control and has a purpose for you in this tragedy."
"Rejoice! God wants to teach you something through your circumstances."

As true as God's Word is and as factual as these statements might be, they can often fail miserably to comfort those who are in pain. Yet it is the context in which these truths are shared, not the content itself, that determines their failure to comfort.

In the aftermath of my recent miscarriage I received several Scripture verses and other spiritual platitudes from well-meaning believers. These people were just trying to help, but their words were very hurtful to me. The fundamental problem was this: Either those who shared their thoughts with me did not know me well enough to know what to say, or they knew me well but were afraid to emotionally connect with me in my grief.

So, in order to play it safe, they distanced themselves from me with propositional truths instead of drawing near to me with incarnational love. Hence, it was not the scriptural truth itself but the way in which the truth was shared that caused me to feel more miserable. I did not sense in those moments that those people truly cared for me. The key here is the quality of relationship. Truth given apart from a loving relationship is not readily received and offers little comfort.

That is why Jesus, who was God incarnate, the embodiment of grace and truth, came to restore a living and vital relationship between God and human beings and not just to relate some ethereal truths about God. Transformation and healing come from a personal, intimate relationship with God, and this relationship is rooted and grounded in the love and forgiveness he offered to us through his Son.

Truth presented in an untimely and insensitive manner can be spiritually and emotionally damaging in and of itself. But truth shared apart from a loving, caring relationship creates more emotional distance between people and further isolates the one who is suffering. This does more to misrepresent the compassionate character of God than anything else!

Someone once told me that "good advice minus a relationship is nothing more than an intrusion." I know that I have sometimes felt intruded upon by sincere believers, as many of you probably have as well. Turning once again to 1 Thessalonians 5:16–18, how do you think the Thessalonian church responded to these statements? Did they view Paul's divinely inspired advice as an intrusion? It's highly unlikely!

Consider, for example, the relational context in which the apostle Paul shared this truth. As we pointed out earlier, he had a deep and abiding relationship with the Thessalonian believers. He cared deeply for them and was well aware of their circumstances. As proof of his love, he sent Timothy to strengthen and encourage them (1 Thess. 3:1–5).

Based on the loving relationship Paul had with these believers and the personal knowledge he had of their desperate situation, he shared the truths found in 1 Thessalonians 5:16–18. He tells them first of all to "rejoice always" (v. 16). The Thessalonians were already filled with joy in spite of severe suffering (1 Thess. 1:6), and Paul also rejoiced in his sufferings (1 Thess. 3:7–9). They were both of one mind. The young church knew that Paul could closely identify with them in their suffering.

To "pray without ceasing" (v. 17) was to constantly acknowledge their dependence upon God. The Lord was to be their strength in the trials they were enduring. Paul was their model in this regard also. In spite of strong opposition, he preached the gospel to the Thessalonians through the strength of his God (1 Thess. 2:2).

In every circumstance they were to give thanks to God (1 Thess. 5:18). Rejoicing, praying, and thanksgiving were just three aspects of God's will for the persecuted Thessalonians, and these are the most difficult things to do in the midst of fiery trials. Yet Paul provided an incarnated pattern for them to follow in this respect as well (1 Thess. 3:9).

The fact that Paul had an intimate relationship with the Thessalonians and could identify with them in their suffering gave credibility to his message. Grace and truth is what he modeled. Though he was imperfect and made mistakes, he genuinely and consistently loved God's people. He left us a timeless and biblical paradigm that should be practiced in the church today.

Through Christ we, too, are capable of speaking the truth in the context of loving and caring relationships. Therefore, we should not harden our hearts against those who have shared with us 1 Thessalonians 5:16–18 or other scriptural truths apart from love and grace, for we have probably done the same thing on occasion. We should embrace the truth they share, knowing that these truths were originally communicated in the context of a loving relationship, with the timeless authority of divine inspiration.

Our goal as disciples of Christ is not to further build emotional walls between one another. We are to break down all barriers and grow together as the body of Christ, accepting each other, including our imperfections, by the grace of God!

11

Building on Recovery and Discipleship

1–2 Timothy and Titus

This is an optimum point in this study of recovery and discipleship across the board in the New Testament to ask and attempt to answer some overarching questions from a scriptural perspective:

1. After the initial, difficult phase of counseling or therapy, what should the next goal be for a Christian in recovery in terms of additional growth (and accountability)?
2. What should a person who has been a disciple for some time have as a longer-term goal for personal growth and ministry?

Before answering, let's clarify the parallel nature of the questions. Both take into account that the *initial phase* of the process (whether recovery or discipleship) should not be expected to go on indefinitely. Both realize that almost any process begins to stagnate if there is not some reasonably clear-cut and obtainable goal to aim for on the path ahead, whether or not all in the process achieve that goal.

The first danger in regard to these related questions is that they not be answered at all. That happens fairly commonly. Believers who thrive in the initial relief and growth of recovery frequently go no further down the road. Having been freed from what had become very much a *discomfort* zone, they find the first comfort zone along the way and settle in for the duration.[1]

It's similar with discipleship. With some new believers, there will be an initial spurt of commitment and growth. After a while, however, it gets to be the "same old, same old" individual discipline and (usually) group dynamics. Sadly, even the life-redirecting nature of discipleship can be reduced to going through the motions!

So it becomes readily apparent that the questions asked above must be answered. We must be cautious, though, because it is so easy to answer them incorrectly.

The Subtle Danger of Half-Baked Answers

You do occasionally hear of cases where the second phase of either recovery or discipleship goes completely awry because of faulty goals or expectations. It is more common, however, to encounter those whose goals are either insufficient or premature.

I know a number of sincere, recovering Christians who set as a growth goal to become a support group leader. With this motivation, they progressed quickly through the recovery process, arriving at the stage in which it was determined that they could take leadership.

At that point, one of two things could be out of kilter:

1. The person involved could be unprepared for the leadership, only appearing to be that stable and far along in the process, often because of the strength of the goal of a leadership role pulling him or her along. In such cases, the person often gets *overwhelmed* and suffers a setback.

2. The person is, in fact, ready for such an initial leadership position, but that kind of position is as far as his or her goal setting ever gets. In that situation, the person *underachieves* and does not progress to the extent that he or she could have.

These two opposite, but equally half-baked, tendencies also occur frequently in a discipleship setting. Premature promotion to leadership often lays disciples low and leaves them fearful of leadership. There are also many truly qualified leaders of first-stage discipleship programs or groups who get stuck at that level, not just in ministry but also in terms of further growth.

In the process of this discussion, it has become clear that the proper goals in both the realms of recovery and discipleship have to do with growth toward leadership. Yet you seldom hear a clear presentation of that process in either realm, much less one with strong biblical moorings. That is what this chapter is about: to attempt at least a first look at the road to leadership for growing believers, whether in recovery or discipleship.

First, however, let's look at a very practical reason why mature, balanced leadership is a necessary goal for believers. What is that pragmatic reason? Supply and demand!

Wanted! Qualified *Super*natural Leaders

Let's face it! True leaders are in great demand, but they are also in disturbingly short supply.

Now, don't jump to a false conclusion here. I did not say that there was a lack of people willing to take leadership (although even that is the case in many ministries). More often than not, one or more strong, natural leaders will emerge to fill the leadership vacuum, either by title or group dynamics.

Therein lies a significant problem in many evangelical ministries. These ministries are frequently started by gifted visionaries, who often are strong, natural leaders. Thus, the embodied conception of leadership that many people in evangelical circles possess is of such a commanding figure.

The rub here is that the Lord is not just looking for leaders, even those who really look and act the part. Rather, he is seeking *super-*

natural leaders—those who are truly scripturally and spiritually qualified for the leadership role.

Otherwise, how can you explain the thrusting of naturally timid Timothy (2 Tim. 1:7), Paul's younger lieutenant, into a key leadership role in the church at Ephesus? Or what about placing an apparently naturally unassuming Titus[2] in a "buzz saw" of ministry on the island of Crete?

This pair are the recipients of the last three New Testament letters that the apostle Paul wrote: 1–2 Timothy and Titus. From these letters we can piece together clues about the latter stages of Paul's life and ministry. We can also sense why the subject of qualified, supernatural leadership was so much on his heart at that point.

Paul's Last Missionary Journey?

At the end of the Book of Acts, Paul was still in jail in Rome (Acts 28:30–31), although the mention of "two full years" likely implies that he was about to be released. Assuming that his release did take place after the statutory limit[3] had come and gone, what happened after that?

In 1 Timothy and Titus, Paul was apparently involved in mobile public ministry, though the circumstances and locations do not fit readily into the narrative of Acts. In 2 Timothy, Paul was in prison, as in the so-called "prison epistles," but in much worse straits, apparently sensing death[4] by execution was near at hand (2 Tim. 4:6–18, 21).

So, the most likely (though obviously not certain) time frame for Paul's grand-finale letters is after the conclusion of Acts (A.D. 61 or 62). Since strong, extrabiblical tradition places Paul's death at the hands of Emperor Nero in A.D. 66 or 67, there would appear to be approximately five years remaining of the apostle's life. Apparently the large majority of that period comprised what could be called "Paul's Fourth (or Last) Missionary Journey."[5]

Getting the (Spiritual) House in Order

Undoubtedly, many things were on Paul's mind during that climactic five-year period of ministry. A priority seemed to be getting his apostolic ministry-related spiritual house in order.

No, I am not so much referring to the details of his own life, although Paul was certainly ready to go and be with the Lord (2 Tim. 4:6–8). Instead, what I have in mind is what the apostle calls "the household of God," the church (1 Tim. 3:15).

Yes, taking the letters of 1–2 Timothy and Titus as the best indication of Paul's ministry priorities during the last phase of his ministry, it appears that establishing adequate qualified, supernatural leadership in the congregations he gave oversight to was near the top of the list. The reasons why that is the case are not difficult to surmise.

First, at least some of the churches had experienced considerable growth and were likely popping at the seams in regard to leadership (including how it was structured; see table 11.1). Thus, they needed apostolic guidance on how to handle such positive growth.

Second, Paul had begun to be convinced that he would not be around indefinitely to offer positive counsel or help correct errors. He needed to put down in writing such guidance to speak to crucial, ongoing issues related to ministry—particularly leadership. After all, it is very rare indeed for a church to rise above the level of the quality of its leadership!

Pastoral Epistles or Leadership Letters?

So far in this chapter, much has been made about 1–2 Timothy being "leadership letters." Perhaps you are wondering why I have not referred to them by their more common moniker—"the Pastoral Epistles."[6]

The reason is that common usage does not make for the best summarization of content. Frankly, it is not completely accurate to say that 1–2 Timothy and Titus are "pastoral letters." That title implies that these three epistles are essentially guidebooks for those in pastoral ministry—at least the way the terminology has been used for much of church history.[7]

Yet such issues take up only a relatively small proportion of these letters. Strictly speaking, neither Timothy[8] nor Titus were pastors. Both were temporary, apostolic representatives—in the turmoil of the church at Ephesus (Timothy) and to the new churches in the hostile, "dysfunctional"[9] environment of Crete (Titus).

So perhaps a better understanding of 1–2 Timothy and Titus is as "leadership letters." After all, both of the named recipients were leaders, as were the elders and deacons they referred to in terms of qualifications and functions (1 Tim. 3, 5; Titus 1). Also, many of the instructions that were given apply to the proper way for leaders to conduct themselves.

Measuring Maturity for People and Churches

One of the hardest things about spiritual leadership is deciding who is really qualified. Often, it comes down to factors of impressiveness of appearance or presentation, when what should be at issue is maturity level.

Paul seemed to understand that frustration. He goes to some lengths to attempt to get beyond the surface and sketch a general attitudinal/behavioral/relational grid for those who are qualified to serve as overseers/elders (Titus 1:5, 7) and deacons (1 Tim. 3:8–13). The characteristics listed are balanced between the primary relationships of life and are not at all a profile that could be met by a prideful, immature person (1 Tim. 3:6).

There are some initially curious features, though, about the differences between the qualifications listed in 1 Timothy 3:1–13 and those in Titus 1:5–9.[10] For example, 1 Timothy deals with both overseers and deacons, while Titus only talks about elders/-overseers.[11] Also, 1 Timothy prohibits a newer disciple from being an overseer, while in Titus he says absolutely nothing about that issue (probably because everyone in the churches on Crete were still new believers). Finally, the teaching qualification in 1 Timothy 3:2 is only one word in the Greek text (*didaktikos*), while it takes twenty-one Greek words to get across the communication qualification in Titus 1:9.

Table 11.1

Church Government in the Pastoral Epistles:
Comparing Positions, Qualifications, and Church Types

Titus 1:5–9	Leadership	1 Timothy 3:1–13	
elder (v. 5), overseer (v. 7) (no deacons mentioned)	positions	overseer (v. 1), elder (5:17)	deacon (vv. 8, 12)
		(full-orbed) Teaching qualifications (v. 2) | not a young believer (v. 6)	
"exhort-refute" qualification (v. 9b)		"exhort-refute" qualification (implied)	
belief" qualification (v. 9a)		"belief" qualification (implied)	"belief" qualification (v. 9)
basic moral-relational qualifications	qualifications for positions	basic moral-relational qualifications	basic moral-relational qualifications
new, smaller churches (Crete)	types of churches	older, larger church(es) (Ephesus)	

Source: Reprinted with permission from A. Boyd Luter, "New Testament Church Government: Fidelity with Flexibility," *Michigan Theological Journal* (fall 1991).

What's the deal? The most simple explanation is that 1 Timothy reflects the qualifications for older, larger churches, while Titus lays out more realistic qualifications for leaders in newer, smaller congregations.

As table 11.1 shows, these complementary qualification lists allow for the growth of both churches and leaders over time. As a church matures, so must the leaders to meet the more challenging qualifications. More leaders (i.e., deacons) are also added to meet the greater needs of the congregation.

These increasingly demanding standards indicate that the Lord is very serious about growing and maturing, even *after* you become a leader. For example, a disciple could qualify to be an overseer/elder by the standards of Titus 1:5–9 but not make it by 1 Timothy 3:1–7.

A key thing to remember here that applies to maturing through both recovery and discipleship is that if you're not going forward, you're not standing still—you're losing ground!

A Recovery-Discipleship Perspective on the Maturity Ladder

Still, there is something that seems very unfair about having leadership and qualifications for leadership as goals that should be placed before recovering and healthy disciples. After all, not everyone can qualify to be in such leadership roles.

Think about it! A brief look at one qualification makes that point. With the "husband of one wife" stipulation for overseers/elders (1 Tim. 3:2; Titus 1:6), women cannot hold that position. If that same phrase is understood in a strict sense, it would also rule out the divorced and the never married as possible elders.

Before concluding that the church's standards for leadership are unfair, however, make a comparison with the ministry of Jesus. Hardly anyone would accuse Christ of unfairness in choosing his twelve apostles from the wider group of disciples (Luke 6:13). Yet, as table 11.2 shows, there are actually proportionately more leaders today than there were in relation to Jesus' ministry. As in Jesus' ministry, there is much more opportunity for

Table 11.2

From Discipleship to Leadership

Context	Initial Status	Progress	Eventual Roles	Proportion
Jesus' ministry	Newer disciples	Growth toward mature discipleship (sanctification; in some cases, recovery)	Apostles (servant/leaders)	Few (12)
			Other key disciples (servants, sometimes leaders, including some women)	Some more
			Other mature disciples, in nonleadership roles	Many
Church ministry			Elders/pastors (servant/leaders)	Relatively few
			Deacons (servants, who also lead on occasion—possibly "deaconesses")	Perhaps more
			Other mature disciples, in non-leadership roles	Many

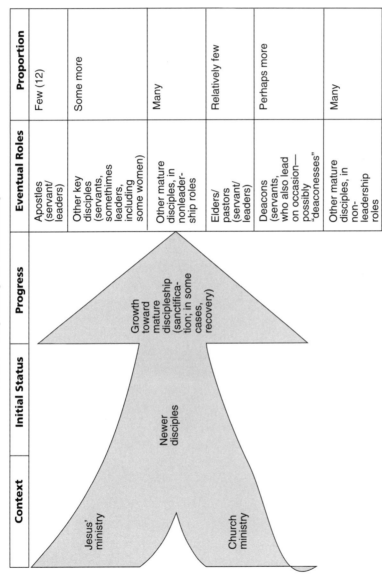

leadership today beyond the "titled" roles—often even if you have really blown it big time in the past! If the maturity and accountability are present, the Lord will provide the context in which to serve, which is what spiritual greatness is all about (Matt. 20:25–28). So, be thankful for whatever opportunities the Lord brings your way. It's icing on the cake if you are allowed to be a servant-leader!

12

Tandem Explorations of Trust Issues

James and Hebrews

In recent times it has become increasingly clear that our culture is in the throes of a crisis of trust. The classic case in point is that polls and other studies consistently reflect that the public in general has less confidence in elected officials and the news media than at any time since studies have been done.

Even more telling, however, is the only slightly greater sense of trust in the educational system and religious institutions. In that regard, you can argue legitimately about the betrayal of public trust especially in the public school and state university systems in the past generation. Likewise, in the religious realm, there have been numerous cults and charlatans in recent years that have tragically abused the trust that was placed in them.

That still does not tell the whole story, however. For many individuals, including a large number of Christians, the lack of trust out there is no more than the tip of the iceberg. They have a very hard time trusting *anyone!*

For many such people, this problem stems from relationships and events in their formative years. Either parents (or guardians) or other crucial natural authority figures during that period in their lives let them down over and over again. Such chronic disappointment breeds distrust, often deep seated.

There are, of course, two sides of the coin on this issue that need to be addressed. This is not simply a problem related to the kind of people (in this case disciples of Jesus Christ) who find it excruciatingly difficult to trust. It is equally, and even more foundationally, a problem of those (far too often believers) who choose not to be trustworthy, especially in their primary relationships (i.e., spouse, children, ministry).

This chapter will deal with both sides. Two New Testament letters, James and Hebrews, combine to address very relevant factors related to both trust and trustworthiness. Thus, these two letters will go hand-in-hand for the purposes of our study.

A Tale of Two Letters

From a recovery/discipleship perspective, the Epistle to the Hebrews deals primarily with restoring faith and trust. In James, on the other hand, the recovery and discipleship focus is on basic faith/trust being translated into a clear-cut visible pattern of trustworthiness.

These letters will be treated in the reverse order of the way they are found in the New Testament for two reasons:

1. James was almost surely written earlier than Hebrews (see table 12.1).
2. Actually, the issue of trust taking feet as consistent trustworthy living (seen in James) is even more basic than developing or reanchoring trust (seen in Hebrews).

In terms of general introduction, James and Hebrews are two of only eight letters in the New Testament that the apostle Paul did not write (although not a few in the church's earlier history have held that Paul did author Hebrews).[1] In both cases, there is not a clearly geographically focused audience being addressed:

James is sent "to the twelve tribes who are dispersed abroad" (1:1);[2] Hebrews gets no more specific than "holy brethren" (3:1; 13:22), though the extensive references to the Old Testament, particularly the Levitical priesthood and its rituals, strongly imply a Jewish readership.[3]

These and other key points that work together from James and Hebrews are summarized in table 12.1. This overview will set up the further recovery/discipleship discussions related to both books.

The major impression to be drawn from this brief, double-barreled survey is that, in a number of important ways, James and Hebrews complement each other's teaching in regard to trust issues. Since James was apparently written earlier, that recognized sequence proves to be a kind of one-two punch about recovery and discipleship—of which we will now sample the force.

James: An Exemplary, Recovering Disciple

It can be confidently concluded that James, the younger half brother of Jesus (Matt. 13:55), is the author of the Book of James. Since he later became, in effect, the longtime senior pastor figure of the Jerusalem church (Acts 15:13–21; 21:17–18), he must be regarded as one of the most prominent Jewish-Christian figures besides the apostles in the New Testament era.[4]

As with Jude, it would have been no picnic growing up in the same household with Jesus. After all, in that case, big brother really was perfect. No younger sibling would come off well in a comparison with Jesus, which likely engendered considerable frustration and resentment.[5]

Perhaps the more difficult thing for James to handle, though, would have been the consecutive losses of his father, Joseph, and then his oldest brother, Jesus, his substitute father figure.[6] From a recovery counseling perspective, it is increasingly clear that the loss or abdication (i.e., often desertion or divorce today) of the crucial father figure at a formative point can be virtually as devastating as a highly abusive father.

Though inferential, it is not at all unlikely that the hesitancy of the younger brothers in Jesus' family to become his disciples (John

Table 12.1
Complementary Angles on Faith

James	Aspects of Comparison	Hebrews
A.D. mid-40s (or early 60s)*	probable date	A.D. later 60s**
Jewish/ knowledgeable of the Old Testament	readers' background	Jewish/ knowledgeable of the Old Testament
trials/ temptation	background issues	past suffering/ present denial
sin and quarrels	response to issues	disillusionment, and backsliding
faith works	angle on trust	faith rests, receives rewards
power of the tongue for abuse or good	focus of structure	Christ, the mediator of the covenant of forgiveness

*Thorough recent evangelical discussions of the dating options related to James can be found in major commentaries such as Peter H. Davids, *Commentary on James*, New International Greek Testament Commentary (Grand Rapids: Eerdmans, 1982); Ralph P. Martin, *James,* Word Biblical Commentary (Waco: Word, 1988); and Douglas J. Moo, *The Letter of James*, Tyndale New Testament Commentaries (Grand Rapids: Eerdmans, 1985). In more compact form, Moo argues persuasively for the mid-40s date over the early 60s position in D. J. Moo, "James," in *Evangelical Commentary on the Bible*, ed. Walter A. Elwell (Grand Rapids: Baker, 1989), 1151; and, most recently, in Carson, Moo, and Morris, *Introduction to the New Testament*, 414.

**Recent substantial conservative discussions of dating alternatives related to Hebrews can be found in F. F. Bruce, *The Epistle to the Hebrews*, rev. ed., New International Commentary on the New Testament (Grand Rapids: Eerdmans, 1990); Donald Guthrie, *The Letter to the Hebrews,* Tyndale New Testament Commentaries (Grand Rapids: Eerdmans, 1983); Donald A. Hagner, *Hebrews*, Good News Commentary (San Francisco: Harper and Row, 1983); and Simon J. Kistemaker, *Exposition of the Epistle to the Hebrews*, New Testament Commentary (Grand Rapids: Baker, 1984). Though lacking certainty, the 60s dating is essentially an evangelical consensus at this point (see Carson, Moo, and Morris, *Introduction to the New Testament*, 400).

7:3) was partly due to feeling this sense of abandonment. The fact that it took a resurrection appearance of Jesus to convince James (1 Cor. 15:7) indicates that his resistance was deep seated.

However, when James did finally become a recovering disciple, he did so with a bang! He was quickly in evidence in the upper room before Pentecost (Acts 1:14). Then, it would not be many years before James's godly lifestyle and leadership ability would earn him the reputation of being a pillar of the church, along with the apostles Peter and John (Acts 12:17; Gal. 2:9). It was out of this pool of recovery/discipleship experience that James's pastor's heart flowed out in letter form to his fellow disciples of Christ (James 2:1).

A Bird's-Eye View of James

There has been no consensus in church history on how to structure the Epistle of James. Moo's studied conclusion is common today: "The letter of James, a series of loosely related homilies, resists clear structural demarcation."[7]

Such is not necessarily the last word on the structure of James, however. The following chiasm seems to legitimately express James's development of thought, as well as highlighting angles of real consequence for recovery and discipleship.

James: A Letter about Trust and Trustworthy Living

A. (1:1–4) Dispersed ones, view trials as a means to grow to maturity
   B. (1:5–8) Receiving wisdom through the prayer of faith
      C. (1:9–18) The temporary nature of wealth, and the blessing and crown for persevering
         D. (1:19–27) Be a doer of the Word who bridles the tongue and is blessed
            E. (2:1–13) It is sinful and lawless for the rich to be partial and merciless, not loving your neighbors
               F. (2:14–26) Faith is displayed by faithful works

G. (3:1–12) The danger of verbal
abuse

F^1. (3:13–18) Wisdom is displayed by
wise behavior

E^1. (4:1–10) It is sinful to be worldly, not
humble, as well as vulnerable to Satan

D^1. (4:11–17) Don't speak against your brother, be
arrogant about God's will, or fail to do the
right thing

C^1. (5:1–12) The rotting of wealth and the need for
patient endurance in light of the Lord's coming

B^1. (5:13–18) Receiving relief and healing through the
prayer of faith

A^1. (5:19–20) Straying ones, view correction as a means to
positive rescue (recovery) and forgiveness[8]

Especially notable here are two points:

1. The outer (A) layer of this structure frames the letter as having to do with the *right* kind of response to difficulties (James 1:2–5) and getting someone back on track after the *wrong* response (5:19–20).
2. The major point at the center of the structure (3:1–12) focuses on the lurking danger and incredible destructiveness of verbal abuse.

The Hebrews: Disciples Sliding into Denial

Relatively little can be known for sure about the background and circumstances of the Jewish readers of the Epistle to the Hebrews but what can be surmised definitely fits well with a recovery/discipleship grid.[9] For example, the force of the first so-called warning passages (Heb. 2:1–4) portrays the pattern of the readers' lives as dangerously adrift (v. 1). Sadly, the current is flowing away from the message and reality of salvation (v. 3) that is the fountainhead of both discipleship and true biblical recovery.

Two more observations related to stern warning passages are also relevant:

1. At least the bulk of the readers had been disciples of Christ long enough to be teachers (5:11–14). Their backsliding represented a major setback in both discipleship and recovery!
2. At some earlier time, the readers had suffered substantially as disciples (10:32–36), and it seems to have had a longer-term disillusioning impact.

Suffice it to say that the Hebrews were turning their backs on Christ, discipleship, and recovery. They were essentially sliding into denial as they flirted more and more with going back into their former legalistic (i.e., spiritually dysfunctional) Jewish lifestyles.

A Bird's-Eye View of Hebrews

The Epistle to the Hebrews is no easier to outline than is James. Unlike James, though, it is "widely agreed that this book has been carefully constructed. What is not agreed is the shape of that structure."[10] In the present climate of uncertainty, it also seems possible that a case can be made for a chiastic structuring.[11] The following outline lays out the parallel thought patterns that reflect such a structure.

Hebrews: A Letter about the Renewal of Trust

A. (1:1–2:18) Christ is superior to the prophets and angels, who serve believing mankind

  B. (3:1–4:13) Christ is superior to Moses and Joshua, but their "rest," sinfully rejected by unbelieving hearts, is still available

    C. (4:14–7:28) Christ is a superior high priest to the priesthood of Aaron, being of the priesthood of Melchizedek

      D. (8:1–13) Christ has a superior ministry because he mediates a better covenant

    C^1. (9:1–10:25) Christ fulfilled the Old Testament worship rituals through his once-for-all sacrifice

  B^1. (10:26–12:29) Christians must live by faith, as exemplary believers always have, putting aside the entanglement of sin, looking ahead to the unshakable kingdom

A[1]. (13:1–25) Christians must live faithfully, by faith, as if entertaining angels[12]

It should especially be noted here that the writer is employing impressive persuasive ability in the attempt to convince the readers that Christ (and his New Covenant) is clearly superior to anything Judaism has to offer and thus a completely worthy object of their trust. Along the way, as the above structure emphasizes (in the B layer), the contrast is stark between the classic examples of the Jews who forfeited so much because of a lack of trust (3:6–4:13) and the Old Testament believers whose faith put them in the "Hall of Fame" (11:1–12:1).

James on Trust: Putting Your Trust to Work

Both James and Hebrews make statements on the nature of trust that apply to discipleship and recovery. It is no coincidence that the almost three-fourths of the focused *faith/trust* terminology in James is found in 2:14–26.[13] Whatever else that long-debated passage may be teaching,[14] it is clearly asserting that true faith will, to some degree, express itself in faithful actions.

What that means for discipleship is that anyone claiming to be a disciple by faith will naturally be expected to present evidence of that discipleship through an exemplary lifestyle of good works. That, by the way, is a point with which Paul is in complete agreement (e.g., Titus 3:8).[15]

What it implies as a principle for recovery is that someone who claims to have (or wants to establish) a trust relationship must display trust*worthy* actions to back up the claim. Otherwise, the desired trusting relationship will be "dead" (James 2:17).

Hebrews on Trust: Salvaging Your Trust after the Depression

As stated previously, it is fairly obvious that Hebrews also has a lot to say about trust[16] and the problem of lack of trust. Let's pay careful attention to both sides of this coin.

First, much of the epistle is taken up with demonstrating what a huge mistake it is to give up on a trust relationship with the most (and only completely) trustworthy person you will ever meet, Jesus. Because of difficult circumstances and following disillusionment, however, that is exactly what the Hebrews were doing.

They were turning and walking away from discipleship and into denial. They were desperately in need of spiritual recovery, and that is what the writer of the Epistle to the Hebrews was trying to bring about!

Second, it's not as if there weren't plenty of positive biblical examples of people who had hung in there in trusting God despite difficult circumstances (Heb. 11). As Hebrews 11:39–40 makes clear, if the readers renew their trust, it will be just as rewarding for them as recovering disciples as was the faith/faithfulness of the Old Testament all-stars.

Please understand, however, that although the Lord is incredibly gracious and loving, "without faith it is impossible to please Him" (11:6). In other words, God is trustworthy, and he is not pleased with those who claim to be stuck at the point of a lack of trust! Thus, there is virtually no legitimate excuse for remaining in a holding pattern very long without progressing in recovery or discipleship.

13

Perspectives of a Recovered Disciple

1–2 Peter

Go away from me, Lord; I am a sinful man! (Luke 5:8).

We have left everything to follow you! (Mark 10:28).

Lord, if it's you, tell me to come to you on the water (Matt. 14:28).

You are the Christ, the Son of the living God (Matt. 16:16).

Never, Lord! This shall never happen to you! (Matt. 16:22).

Even if I have to die with you, I will never disown you (Matt. 26:35).

I don't know the man! (Matt. 26:74).

Yes, Lord, you know that I love you (John 21:15).

Therefore let all Israel be assured of this: God has made this Jesus, whom you crucified, both Lord and Christ (Acts 2:36).

To the elders among you, I appeal as a fellow elder, a witness of Christ's sufferings and one who also will share in the glory to be revealed (1 Peter 5:1).

To him be glory both now and forever! Amen (2 Peter 3:18).

All quotations are from NIV

J esus said that the things that flow out of a person's mouth come from the heart (Matt. 15:18). The words of Simon Peter quoted above clearly manifest the many facets of his heart. They also brilliantly reveal the progress he made on his discipleship and recovery journey.

His path was an extraordinarily bumpy one, full of twists and turns. It seemed as though he was consistently taking two steps forward and three steps back. But by the grace of his Lord, Simon finally lived up to his divinely given name, Peter. He became a rock (*Peter* literally means *rock*)—an immovable pillar of faith.

Because so many of us can identify with Peter's experience, we are going to look more closely at his life. In this respect, this chapter will be slightly different from the others, but it will prove to be a valuable study, because Peter's epistles profoundly reflect the lessons he learned in the school of Christ.

Therefore, before we delve into the content of his letters, we will give a brief overview of the life of Simon Peter, a man with an impetuous, yet sincere, heart.

Snapshots of Simon Peter in the Gospels

Simon was originally from Bethsaida (John 1:44), a city in Galilee located on the west coast of the Sea of Galilee. He and his brother, Andrew, made their home in Capernaum, which was also located on the western shore of the Sea of Galilee (Mark 1:29). Simon and Andrew were fishermen by trade and, considering where they lived, they probably had a fairly successful business.

Christ found Simon and his brother casting their nets into the Sea of Galilee and called them to follow him. They immediately left everything and became his disciples (Matt. 4:18–20; Mark 1:16–18; Luke 5:1–11). Simon, along with James and John, the sons of Zebedee, were Christ's closest companions and disciples. We commonly refer to the three of them as "the inner circle."

Not long after his initial calling, Simon was designated an apostle (Matt. 10:2; Mark 3:16; Luke 6:14). He is always placed first in the listings of the twelve apostles and also wherever the inner circle is specifically named (Mark 5:37). Simon was the first to confess Jesus as Christ (Matt. 16:16; Mark 8:29; Luke 9:20), and it is to him that Jesus gives the keys to the kingdom of heaven (Matt. 16:18–19).[1]

It is in the context of this confession that Jesus decisively changed Simon's name to *Peter*, the rock. This is the first indication of what he was to become under the tutelage and guidance of his Master. Yet what Jesus had to work with also becomes clear as Simon's rash and impetuous nature increasingly manifested itself.

Simon Peter was the only disciple to openly rebuke Jesus. He did this not once but on at least three occasions:

1. when Jesus foretold his persecution and death (Matt. 16:21–23)
2. when the crowds were pressing against Jesus and the sick woman touched him (Luke 8:45)
3. when he refused to let Jesus wash his feet (John 13:6–11)

Simon Peter is specifically named as witnessing the miracles of Jesus and as being present during many of the key events in Jesus' life:

1. Jesus enabled him to walk on the water of the Sea of Galilee (Matt. 14:28–31).
2. He was present at the healing of Jairus's daughter (Mark 5:37).
3. He was present at the transfiguration (Matt. 17:1–8; Mark 9:2–8; Luke 9:28–36).
4. He was present at the Garden of Gethsemane (Matt. 26:36–46; Mark 14:33–42; Luke 22:40–46).

5. He followed Jesus to the high priest's palace (Matt. 26:58; Mark 14:54; Luke 22:54; John 18:15).

On several occasions, Simon Peter proved himself eager to learn his Master's ways. He specifically sought the interpretation of the parable of the manager (Luke 12:41), of the law of forgiveness (Matt. 18:21), of the law of defilement (Matt. 15:15), and of the second coming (Mark 13:34).

Clearly, the low point of Simon Peter's life came in his three-fold denial of Jesus (Matt. 26:69–75; Mark 14:66–72; Luke 22:55–62; John 18:17–18, 25–27)—the event for which he is most well-known. What undoubtedly made this event even more painful for Simon was that he had previously sworn unswerving allegiance to Jesus (Matt. 26:33–35)! Overcome by grief, he went out from the Lord's presence and wept bitterly (Luke 22:61–62).

John 21 shows that the Lord Jesus completely forgave Simon Peter and reinstated him into the ranks of ministry. Jesus also revealed to Simon the kind of death he would die in order to glorify God (John 21:18–19). However, it does not seem from this context that he was yet ready to make this sacrifice (John 21:20–21).

With the closing of the Book of John and the opening of the Book of Acts, an amazing transformation begins to take place in the life of Simon Peter. The new Peter emerges. The coming of the Holy Spirit ushers Peter to a deeper phase in his discipleship and recovery process.

From Simon to Peter: The Book of Acts

To go from the Book of John to the Book of Acts is a simple turn of the page. But what a difference a page makes! Christ gave Peter his new name, and with the coming of the Holy Spirit in Acts 2, Peter began to live up to his name. By grace, the Lord had successfully molded and shaped Simon into Peter. Lockyer gives further insight into this incredible transformation:

"Thou art . . . Thou shall be." Was this not an evidence of our Lord's omniscience? Here was an insight penetrating to the deepest recesses of Simon Peter's nature, and a wisdom revealing that He

could not expect more from Peter than he could give, but also a faith that once all the angularities of his character had been rounded off, he would be a vessel unto honor. Thus it was love that bore with Peter's limitations as he emerged from his old life. Grace pardoned his failures, and he became an apostle to leave the impact of utter devotion to Christ upon succeeding ages. The latent possibilities under the surface of Peter's nature, then, were read by Christ with prophetic insight into a forecast of his true character, and the new name of Cephas or Peter, He gave him was the first lash of divine inspiration in the ministry of Christ.[2]

After the ascension of his Lord, Peter remained in Jerusalem (Acts 1:13). He was the one who suggested to the other apostles that someone be elected to fill Judas's place (Acts 1:15–22). After the Holy Spirit descended on those in the upper room, Peter was the first to preach the good news to those gathered in Jerusalem for Pentecost (Acts 2:14–40).

Peter was clearly the spokesman for the other apostles. When they were all accused by the council of wrongdoing, he was the one to stand before the council and make a defense (Acts 4:1–23; 5:17–42). He was also the first one to mete out judgment in the church by foretelling the deaths of Ananias and Sapphira (Acts 5:1–11).

The preaching of the gospel to the Samaritans was made complete by Peter when they received the Holy Spirit by the laying on of his hands (Acts 8:14–17). He was also the first to preach the gospel to the Gentiles (Acts 10) and, in the context of the Jerusalem council (Acts 15), was one of the first to advocate preaching the gospel to the Gentiles.

Peter, just like his Lord before him, performed extraordinary miracles by the power of the Holy Spirit:

1. healing of the crippled man in the portico of the temple (Acts 3:1–10)
2. healing of the paralytic, Aeneas (Acts 9:32–34)
3. raising Dorcas from the dead (Acts 9:36–43)

These are just a few of the specifically recorded miracles, but it is clear that he performed many more (Acts 5:15).

Much more could be said about Peter, but what has been said is enough to show just how incredibly prominent he is in the Gospels and the Book of Acts. In fact, apart from the Lord Jesus, there is no one mentioned more often in the Gospels than Peter. It is an amazing thing that the disciple we can identify with the most is the one who is most talked about in the New Testament.

This is certainly no accident. God intended for us to learn much about him and ourselves through the life and experiences of this man. As we have seen through our brief survey of Peter's words and deeds, discipleship and recovery did not come easy for him at first.

However, as the Book of Acts has shown and as his two epistles will further reveal, he did eventually learn from his experiences in the school of Christ. The Lord was able to bring this big fisherman to a level of spiritual maturity that Peter himself probably didn't think was possible. We will explore this angle of his discipleship and recovery in the remainder of this chapter.

Before we move on, however, we should deal with one more issue concerning Peter's spiritual growth. You might be tempted to think that Peter had an advantage over us because he walked with Jesus and interacted with him face-to-face. After all, he was able to see and experience firsthand Jesus' power to change lives. That must be why Peter's discipleship and recovery were such a success.

I would like to point out, though, that Peter's eyewitness of Christ's miracles and the personal contact he had with Christ ultimately did not change his heart. He did not fully understand, at that point, the sacrifice and commitment involved in being one of Christ's disciples. If Peter had understood it, he probably would not have denied his Lord.

If walking with Christ face-to-face did not change Peter, then what did? It was the indwelling Holy Spirit and a life of walking in the Spirit that made the supreme difference. It was *faith* that brought about spiritual and emotional maturity in Peter. It was learning to trust in the God whom he could not see that caused his growth.

In his book *Disappointment with God*, Philip Yancey talks with unusual wisdom and insight about God's desire to have a mature people. As the history of Israel in the Old Testament clearly shows, God's physical presence in the pillar of clouds did not produce this maturity. In fact, it did quite the opposite. The Israelites became increasingly more rebellious, hardened, and unbelieving.

Hence, Israel's and Peter's history essentially prove that God's physical presence does not guarantee spiritual and emotional maturity. Only faith can produce this kind of growth. And God has been moving his people to faith since his calling of Abraham (Gen. 12). Here, at the end of the ages, God has accomplished his goal by sending the Holy Spirit to indwell his people. We, like Peter, belong to the age of the Spirit—the age of faith.

God's unseen presence by the Holy Spirit makes faith necessary and, therefore, makes maturity a real possibility. In a section entitled, "A Trinity of Voices," Yancey points out how God has worked out his plan to bring his people to maturity:

> Think of God's plan as a series of Voices. The first Voice, thunderingly loud, had certain advantages. When the Voice spoke from the trembling mountain at Sinai, or when fire licked up the altar on Mount Carmel, no one could deny it. Yet, amazingly, even those who heard the Voice and feared it—the Israelites at Sinai and at Carmel, for example—soon learned to ignore it. Its very volume got in the way. Few of them sought out that Voice; fewer still persevered when the Voice fell silent.
>
> The Voice modulated with Jesus, the *Word* made flesh. For a few decades the Voice of God took on the timbre and volume and rural accent of a country Jew in Palestine. It was a normal human voice, and though it spoke with authority, it did not cause people to flee. Jesus' voice was soft enough to debate against, soft enough to kill.
>
> After Jesus departed, the Voice took on new forms. On the day of Pentecost, tongues—*tongues*—of fire fell on the faithful, and the church, God's body, began to take shape. That last Voice is as close as breath, as gentle as a whisper. It is the most vulnerable Voice of all, and the easiest to ignore. The Bible says the Spirit can be "quenched" or "grieved." . . . Yet the Spirit is the most intimate Voice. . . . The Spirit whispers of a new reality, a fantasy that is actually true, one into which we will awake for eternity.[3]

For three years, Peter personally walked with Jesus, the second Voice of the Trinity. But it was during the thirty years that he walked *by faith* with the Holy Spirit, the unseen third Voice of the

Trinity, that he truly blossomed and matured. The many lessons Peter learned during that time are preserved for us in his two Spirit-inspired letters.

1 Peter and 2 Peter

It is most profitable to compare the portrait of Peter in the gospels and his pronouncements in his epistles. How amazingly and gloriously different they are! In the gospels, Peter had the privilege of seeing his Lord transfigured; in his epistles, Peter is before us transfigured by the matchless, boundless grace of God.

In the gospels, we see Peter impetuous, courageous, quick to meet personal slight, ambitious of earthly power, self-confident yet cowardly.

In his epistles, we see Peter subdued, patient, forbearing, humble, loving, with all his old buoyancy and courage purified and enobled.[4]

The apostle Peter wrote his epistles to meet the pressing needs of believers, both Jew and Gentile alike, who were undergoing a terrible time of suffering and persecution. These Christians were scattered throughout northern Asia Minor (modern Turkey), which was a vast region of the Roman Empire (1 Peter 1:1–2).[5]

These letters clearly reflect Peter's pastoral heart. They are filled with statements of encouragement, exhortation, and warning designed to spur believers on to maturity and holy living. The major themes of faith, suffering, and maturity particularly relate to discipleship and recovery.

Faith

The following verses show the prominence of the theme of faith. The suffering the saints were enduring had come so that their faith might be purified and refined (1 Peter 1:7a, 9). Faith is of greater worth than gold and must be proved genuine at the coming of the Lord (1 Peter 1:7b), and suffering is the tool God uses to prove our faith.

In 2 Peter, Christians are to express their faith by believing God's prophetic and written Word (2 Peter 1:4, 16–17, 19; 3:2, 5, 7, 9,

13, 15). Believers must put their faith in God's Word in order not to be deceived by false teachers (2 Peter 2).

Suffering

This is considered the most prominent theme running through the Book of 1 Peter. According to Wiersbe, Peter recalls the sufferings of Christ in order to encourage persecuted believers and also to show how suffering is closely linked to grace and glory.

> One of the encouragements that Peter gives suffering saints is the assurance that their suffering will one day be transformed into glory (1:6–7; 4:13–14; 5:10). This is possible only because the Saviour suffered for us and then entered into His glory (1:11; 5:1). The sufferings of Christ are mentioned often in this letter (1:11; 3:18; 4:1, 13; 5:1).
>
> But suffering does not automatically bring glory to God and blessing to God's people. . . . It is only when we depend on the grace of God that we can glorify God in times of suffering. The word "grace" is used in every chapter of 1 Peter. . . . Whatever begins with God's grace will always lead to glory.[6]

Peter was an eyewitness of Christ's sufferings and undoubtedly underwent much suffering himself during his years of ministry. He learned to value suffering for Christ's sake because of the spiritual fruit it produced in his life.

Hence, one of the major points Peter makes in his first epistle is that suffering is an essential part of the Christian life and is actually necessary for our faith and maturity. He also holds up Christ as the ultimate example of suffering for the glory of God (1 Peter 2:20–25).

When we consider who Peter was when Christ first met him on the shores of the Galilee, it is amazing that these kinds of revelations could flow from his pen. This is the same man who rebuked his Lord for even talking about suffering (Matt. 16:22)!

However, Peter learned well from Christ's example that suffering according to God's will is indeed one of the highest callings for the Christian (1 Peter 4:19). Suffering will bring us to spiritual maturity if we allow it to.

Maturity

Naturally, spiritual and emotional maturity is a great concern of Peter's. In his first epistle, he encourages believers to express maturity by holy living (1 Peter 1:13–25) and by doing good deeds (1 Peter 2:12; 3:13). They were to live such good lives among the pagans that even they would glorify God (2:12)! This they were to do in spite of severe persecution.

In 2 Peter, the call to maturity comes not so much as an encouragement but more as a stern warning. Believers were to make every effort to grow in Christian virtues in order to make their calling and election sure (2 Peter 1:5–10). In other words, if they were not growing, maybe they should begin to question if they really belonged to Christ!

Spiritual growth was one way the Christians in the first century could be assured of their salvation. This is also a strong warning to all of Christ's disciples in every age. According to the apostle Peter, spiritual maturity should be taken very seriously and should be hotly pursued.

In this matter, discipleship and recovery dovetail beautifully. To mature as a disciple of Christ is to take a giant step forward in the recovery process. In fact, it could be said that the extent of our recovery is directly related to our maturity as a disciple.

In the context of his discussion concerning the events surrounding the second coming of Christ, Peter asks this pointed question: "Since everything will be destroyed in this way, what kind of people ought you to be?" His answer? "You ought to live holy and godly lives" (2 Peter 3:11 NIV).

For Peter, then, the second coming of Christ is also a solid motivation to pursue maturity. We don't often think of the second coming of Christ as being an incentive to grow up in the Lord. Instead, we think of it primarily as a time of great woe for unbelievers. But Peter's warning to *believers* in this context is very clear. In fact, his last recorded words have to do with this need for maturity: "But grow in the grace and knowledge of our Lord and Savior Jesus Christ" (2 Peter 3:18 NIV). This will safeguard us against false teaching (v. 17) and assure us that we are at peace with him (3:14).

Peter was a man whom the Lord tamed, recovered, and then transformed into a humble, gracious disciple. The things Peter learned from his personal encounter with Christ and from years of walking with him by faith have come down to us as timeless biblical truths pertinent to both discipleship and recovery.

14

The Gnostic Error and Recovery

1-3 John

When the apostle John wrote his Gospel, he clearly stated his purpose and goal: "These have been written that you may believe that Jesus is the Christ, the Son of God; and that believing you may have life in His name" (John 20:31). While his purpose is clear, the theological concepts developed in his book are most profound and sometimes difficult to understand. A beginner could certainly benefit from reading John's Gospel, but it would take an avid student to adequately plunge the depths of its meaning.

Many of the same penetrating insights and theology permeate the epistles that bear his name. First John is especially complex in style, structure, and thought, but it is not so far beyond ready comprehension as to confuse the average reader. On the contrary, it is the straightforwardness of its message that will convict the heart and shape the character of every willing believer.

This paradoxical combination of theologically complex and essentially straightforward themes is John's trademark and is evident throughout his writings. For instance, 1, 2, and 3 John are filled with exhortations to continue in the truth and to beware of those who have strayed from it (see 1 John 2:24, 26; 3:7; 4:4–6; 5:19–21; 2 John 9–10; 3 John 3, 9–11). This is the clear and basic message of these letters. The complexity is found in some of the concepts and metaphors John uses to communicate the essence of true Christianity (see 1 John 1:1–3, 6–7; 2:6, 27; 3:9; 4:15; 5:6–10).

Truth or Dire Consequences

Because of the infiltration of false teachers into the late first century churches, the apostle wrote his first letter to help believers discern truth from error. These teachers were threatening the peace of the Christian communities by spreading erroneous doctrine. Schisms and divisions began to develop as some believers were being drawn away from the fold to follow after these men.[1]

John eloquently attacked these false teachers by reaffirming the true nature of Christianity and by clarifying the nature of the doctrinal errors of these men. Admittedly, there is some debate among evangelical scholars concerning the identity of these false teachers or whether John was refuting false teachers at all. However, most would generally agree that he was indeed warring against fallacious teachers and that the doctrine they were presenting was some early (incipient) form of Gnosticism.[2]

Glenn Barker refers to John's unusual approach to dealing with this heresy and discusses the significance of his epistles throughout church history:

> If John's epistles address the problem of heresy, they do so in unconventional terms. They insist that true Christian faith requires knowing that Jesus the Christ came in human flesh, lived a human life, and died in the flesh. But the evidence of that faith is measured by the genuineness of one's Christian lifestyle, not so much by what one "knows." The knowledge that God is light is tested by whether one walks in that light and obeys God's commands. The knowledge that God is righteous is tested by whether one lives righteously as befits one born of God. The knowledge that God is love is tested by whether one loves fellow believers even as one loves God. The single but radical requirement for love and obedience in the Johannine Epistles recalls the simplicity of Jesus' own

teaching and the radical response he required of those who would follow him. The ability of these letters to recall to the church its origins and cause it to hear afresh the word of him who came in the flesh has preserved a special place for them in the life and devotion of the church.[3]

This poignant description of the purpose of John's letters beckons us in the twentieth century to rediscover and apply the truths found in them. It is in this context of warning and exhortation that we must understand the argument of his epistles, for it appears that the late first century believers were in a serious predicament. They were apparently being preyed upon by false shepherds, and the truth they had learned and believed in was being called into question.

The apostle John exploded the fallacious teachings of the Gnostics with each stroke of his pen. By giving the churches exact criteria to know whether or not they were walking in the truth, he brilliantly exposed the Gnostics' doctrinal errors. John accomplished two timeless objectives in his impassioned approach:

1. He taught believers to discern truth from error by reaffirming what is true.
2. He solemnly warned them to live in the light of the truth they have received.

As Barker pointed out, one of the vital points John makes in his epistles is that spiritual truth has practical implications. As believers, we are personally responsible to live in accordance with the truth revealed to us in the Scriptures.

It is in the apostle John's battle for spiritual and personal truth that we find application for discipleship and recovery. The early Gnostic error reaches down through the centuries and subtly impacts us today, sowing seeds of dissension and dividing the church along enemy lines. Therefore, a clear understanding of the Gnostic problem is needed in order to fully apply the message of 1–3 John.

The Gnostic Split

In their book, *False Assumptions*, Henry Cloud and John Townsend discuss the problem of the Gnostic split. They attempt to expose the error of what they call "sufficiency teaching" by showing its relation to this ancient heresy. In order to understand the full impact of Cloud and Townsend's argument, I've included their complete discussion on the subject from their book:

> At the root of sufficiency teaching is Gnosticism, an ancient philosophy that held that knowledge of spiritual things is essential. Matter—the opposite of spirit—is therefore evil. In other words, flesh is bad and spirit is good. The goal of the Gnostic, then, was to become less fleshly and more spiritual.
>
> It was only logical that Gnostics treated their bodies, which were matter, harshly. Self-mutilation, deprivation, and isolation were commonly practiced by them, all to help Gnostics separate their flesh from their spirit. Their view of Christ? A purely spiritual Christ, not one tainted by humanity.
>
> With the opening words of his first letter, John explodes this heresy. . . . The apostle's point was that the Christ was also a man named Jesus, who lived, breathed, touched us, and died for us. In the same way he loved us, we are to love others. The spiritual Christian is very, very human.
>
> For this reason, the phrase "body of Christ" is critically important. In passages like Romans 12, 1 Corinthians 12, and Ephesians 4 we read that the church operates as Jesus' body would if he were physically still on earth. We are to love each other, bear each other's burdens, and support each other. We are his fingers.[4]

Cloud and Townsend's point on the error of the Gnostic split is well taken. They aptly demonstrate how the false assumption, "If I have God, I don't need people," can be traced back to the Gnostics' interpretation of the distinction between good (spirit) and evil (matter). This doctrine has indeed been kept alive by some teachers in the evangelical church today and, as Cloud and Townsend attest, manifests itself by downplaying our need for each other.

They quote the Pauline phrase "body of Christ" in order to support the biblical truth that we do in fact need each other and are commanded to love and support one another. However, it is not the apostle Paul who explodes the heresy of the Gnostic split but John who completely demolishes this teaching.

Cloud and Townsend rightly point out in their argument that "with the opening words of his first letter, John explodes" the Gnostics' heretical splitting of the nature of Christ. In fact, John's entire letter deals with how this teaching affects our behavior and our relationships to one another—that is, how it opposes the truth. For that reason, throughout his epistle John overwhelmingly demonstrates our need to love and support one another. In fact, John says to *not* love each other is to "walk in darkness" and not live by the truth (1 John 2:9–11).

The Gnostics, who split Christ's nature (thus denying the incarnation), ultimately undermined love and truth, two characteristics essential to discipleship and the recovery process. As we have seen, this dangerous Gnostic teaching still lurks among us today. Besides downplaying our need for human relationships, what is known in recovery circles as the "psychological split" between the "all-good" you and the "all-bad" you could also be considered another manifestation of this heresy. Therefore, we must be careful not to falsely dichotomize our own nature, as the Gnostics did to Christ's. We are fallen and sinful creatures, but we are not completely consumed by evil.[5]

Nevertheless, it must be pointed out that not all splitting is bad. For instance, there are some crucial black-and-white distinctions that must be made when dealing with biblical theology. A crucial example is the difference between truth and error. These two concepts play an important role in both discipleship and recovery. John brought truth and error into sharp focus as he battled the Gnostic belief system.

The Legitimate Split

Before we go any further, it must be understood that Gnosticism did not become a full-blown belief system until the second century. As it has been clearly seen from John's epistles, however, some of its basic tenets were being formed in the latter part of the first century and posed a great threat to the orthodox Christian faith.[6]

John was deeply concerned that his readers be grounded in the truth so that they might not be deceived by teachers who embraced this early Gnostic error. Curtis Vaughan briefly described in more detail the basic principles of early Gnosticism, which gives us further insight into the polemics of John's epistles:

> (1) [Gnosticism] made knowledge, not faith, the one condition of salvation and the only test of fellowship with God. This knowledge, however, was not open to everyone but was the privilege only of those who had been initiated into the mysteries of the Gnostic system. It was therefore an esoteric knowledge to which simple believers could not attain. This distorted emphasis on knowledge led to arrogance, lovelessness, and exclusivism. It also gave the movement its name, the Greek word for knowledge being *gnosis*.
>
> (2) It taught that all matter is inherently evil. This doctrine, in turn, led the Gnostics into at least two other very grave errors, one practical and the other theological. The *practical* error concerned the nature of the Christian life. Starting with the assumption that the body is evil, some Gnostics turned to asceticism and others to the opposite extreme of licentiousness. . . .
>
> *Theologically*, the Gnostic belief in the inherent evil of matter led to an outright denial of the real Incarnation of God in Christ. . . . Every sentence of 1 John reflects the apostle's abhorrence of the Gnostic system. He taught that it was wholly subversive of Christianity and that no compromise whatsoever could be made with it.[7]

The apostle John made it clear that any compromise with the Gnostics would jeopardize the truth. What is of interest to us here is the Gnostics' emphasis on knowledge. To them, knowledge was salvation, and only a few could attain it. As Vaughan pointed out, this belief ultimately brought forth bad fruit. The pursuit of knowledge as an end in itself produced pride, arrogance, and exclusivism.

Many believers in the first century were deeply hurt by those who embraced this exclusivistic idea of knowledge and salvation, and there are Christians today who have been left out by those who hold to this same error. These bewildered believers are plagued with feelings of inferiority. Because they can never quite measure up to others in the area of knowledge, it seems as though they are always on the outside looking in.

It's not that knowledge itself is the culprit here. It is the *motivation* behind the pursuit of knowledge that can often cause this kind of problem. Knowledge is not inherently evil, nor is it directly responsible for division and strife. There is, however, such a thing as *bad* knowledge—knowledge that produces evil; a knowledge of falsehood that can destroy harmonious relationships.

That is why there can be a legitimate need to split; there is a good reason to draw the line between certain things. In this case, the legitimate split comes between knowledge of the truth and knowledge of the false. The Gnostics strived for knowledge and saw it as a means of salvation. Their pursuit was based on the false assumption that knowledge saves a person. Those who embraced knowledge for this reason, a knowledge of falsehood, produced bad fruit (arrogance, pride, broken relationships).

Knowledge of truth, however, brings forth good fruit. John admonishes believers to walk in the truth they have come to know through him (1 John 1:1–5). Knowledge of the truth is vitally important to John. He uses the word *know* (Greek *ginōskō*) thirty-eight times in his epistles. That is more than any other New Testament writer. According to the apostle, we are to pursue and practice the knowledge of the truth.

No one is ever excluded from this pursuit. Every believer can attain to the knowledge of the truth. Therefore, the ultimate legitimate split is between the truth and the false—not between people. Cloud and Townsend pointed out that the Gnostic split between matter (evil) and spirit (good) undermined unity and downplayed our need for each other. Vaughan also affirmed how this belief denies the incarnation of Christ, erroneously splitting him into the man Jesus and the divine Christ.

The truth is that we are all basically on level ground when it comes to pursuing the knowledge of God. He does not split people into categories according to their intellect, giving more knowledge of himself to those who appear to be mentally superior. Knowledge of the truth is not reserved for those who are smart by the standards of this world. It is available to everyone, and we are all commanded to pursue it. This knowledge of the truth is expressed by loving God and loving one another.

Whether we are aware of it or not, we have all been affected by the ancient Gnostic heresy to one degree or another. The degree to which it has influenced us, of course, depends on many factors. If you have been in intimate contact with someone who has knowingly or unknowingly embraced Gnostic beliefs, then you probably have experienced some of the things we have been discussing.

You may have been left out of the "in" crowd and feel that you do not measure up. There is a good chance that you have been taught that your human part is bad and your spiritual part is all that matters, that human relationships are good, but not necessary if you have the Lord.

John's message is highly relevant to all who have endured this kind of treatment. He teaches us that there is a legitimate split to be considered: The split is between good and evil, between truth and error. The erroneous Gnostic belief, which splits people apart and fragments the personality, should be avoided at all costs! The apostle warns us to stay away from those who teach these things and to stand firm in the truth.

At the heart of both discipleship and recovery is this relentless pursuit of the truth. John points out that knowledge of the truth, especially as it pertains to the incarnation of Christ, is an essential part of the Christian life. He precisely informs us what this truth means and how it should be lived out on a daily basis. The apostle solemnly warns us that our true identity will ultimately be revealed by our actions.

Practicing the Truth

To sum up all we have been discussing in this chapter concerning the Gnostic error and recovery, we will refer directly to John's first epistle. He vividly describes how we can know God, who is the Truth, and how our knowledge of him must be expressed by love and obedience. The key foundation on which his letter is built is the incarnation of Christ.

As Cloud, Townsend, and Vaughan previously pointed out, the Gnostics adamantly denied the incarnation, which necessarily distorted other key aspects of salvation (e.g., the atonement, resurrection). Because of this, John began his letter with his own personal testimony of the incarnation. He invited his readers to fellowship with him, and he attested that his fellowship was with the Father and his Son, Jesus Christ (1 John 1:1–4).

John's overriding focus was on the tender mercy of God, who faithfully demonstrated his love through the sacrifice of his Son. The beloved apostle also testified that those who are of the truth, who are the true children of God, must follow Christ's example by expressing this same kind of sacrificial love. The truth of the incarnation is echoed throughout his letter, striking deadly blows to the Gnostic denial of this foundational doctrine.

It is not difficult to see the connection between John's flow of thought and discipleship and recovery. Truth, love, and obedience—three biblical concepts manifested in the incarnation and critical to John in refuting the Gnostics—are very relevant to both discipleship and recovery. Recovering disciples who know and practice God's truth are less likely to be influenced and torn apart by lies rooted in Gnosticism.

Therefore, it would be a great benefit to us all to understand the careful progression of John's argument against those who deny the incarnation. The divinely inspired chiastic structure of his letter brilliantly reveals his overall purpose to correct this false teaching and encourage disciplined living.

A. (1:1–4) John's testimony: The Word of Life appeared (*the reality of the incarnation*) and has offered fellowship with himself and his Father.

  B. (1:5–2:17) God is light. We must walk with him in the light and love one another as he commanded us (*the expression of the incarnation*).

    C. (2:18–27) Beware of antichrists who deny the Father and the Son (*the denial of the incarnation*).

      D. (2:28–3:24) Children of God must love each other as he commanded. Jesus Christ is our supreme example of sacrificial love (*the reality and expression of the incarnation*).

    C¹. (4:1–6) Beware of the spirit of antichrist who denies that Jesus Christ has come in the flesh *(denial of the incarnation)*.

   B¹. (4:7–5:5) God is love. We should walk in love as he commanded us *(the expression of the incarnation)*.

A¹. (5:6–21) God's testimony: the Spirit, the water, and the blood *(the reality of the incarnation)*. God has given us eternal life in his Son. We know him who is true, and we are in him who is true.

Each mirroring idea supports and affirms the incarnation of Christ. It is the crux of John's argument against the Gnostic heresy. When this vital doctrine is compromised, the rest of the Christian faith falls to pieces. The incarnation of Christ is a living reality that must be applied to the life of the recovering disciple. It is the relentless pursuit of the knowledge of the truth that merges the paths of discipleship and recovery together.

15

Concluding the Great Commission and Recovery

Revelation

Stereotypes can be very damaging. They highlight certain features out of proportion to their importance and essentially overlook others that may be just as important, though not as obvious. In so doing, they leave a lopsided and, hence, distorted perspective.

The Book of Revelation has been stereotyped by many people as focusing almost exclusively on the judgments of the wrath of God at the end of the age, just before the second coming of the Lord Jesus Christ. That, of course, is basically correct . . . as far as it goes. There is, however, much more to Revelation than judgment.

It will be amazing to such people that Revelation has anything to say about the subjects of recovery[1] and discipleship. It will be absolutely astounding to think that it has a great deal to say! Yet you don't have to proceed very far in the Apocalypse to make both connections.

The Book of Revelation serves, in effect, as the conclusion of the New Testament.[2] Accordingly, this chapter will explore Revelation for the concluding angles on recovery and discipleship seen in the New Testament. Then the epilogue will provide a brief conclusion for the entire volume, summarizing in three tables the broad directions of New Testament teaching in both areas.

John's Angle on Overcoming Intense Suffering

In Revelation 1:9, the apostle John[3] is on the island of Patmos, apparently as a prisoner. He states that the reasons for his incarceration were "the word of God and the testimony of Jesus." John has also been suffering *tribulation* (Greek *thlipsis*) to some extent, as have at least some of his readers (v. 9).

For John, suffering at the hands of abusive power figures was nothing new. He had watched Jesus suffer unjustly at the hands of the Jewish and Roman leaders as apparently the only male disciple at the foot of the cross ("the disciple whom He loved," John 19:26–27).[4] He had been an innocent victim of Jewish persecution during much of the period narrated in the first half of Acts. He may well have even experienced some of the Roman onslaught prior to the destruction of Jerusalem in A.D. 70.

The key point here is: John *knew* tribulation! He knew painful suffering better than Bo Jackson ever knew a sport! He was eminently qualified to record the visions of the Book of Revelation, which portray the worst tribulation[5] of history.

This perspective is incredibly valuable because John's personal experience and the inspired scriptural content of Revelation combine to confidently state that it is possible to stand firm as an overcomer no matter what level of undeserved suffering comes your way. This is great news on both the recovery and discipleship fronts!

From a commitment standpoint, *overcoming* is very much a term of discipleship, but it is no less a recovery term. To be an overcomer is to emerge from undeserved abuse and suffering a spiritual winner, not a lifelong victim.

It is even very plausible to overview the entire Apocalypse from the yoked perspectives of recovery and discipleship, as can be seen in table 15.1:

Table 15.1
A Recovery/Discipleship Outline of Revelation

I. chapter 1	Suffering overshadowed by the glory of Christ
II. chapters 2–3	The churches in denial and discipleship
III. chapters 4–5	The heavenly focal point of discipleship and recovery
IV. chapters 6–16	Waning opportunity to repent and the intensifying divine judgments
V. chapters 17–19	Just, destructive consequences of standing against God
VI. chapter 20	Face-to-face with the Lord, but denial still occurs
VII. chapters 21–22	Eternal discipleship beyond sin and recovery

Adapted from Luter, "Revelation," in *Life Recovery Bible,* 1449.

The Church in Microcosm: Wrestling with Recovery and Discipleship

Taking a closer look at the most obviously relevant and applicable portion of the Book of Revelation reveals a similar intertwining of these pillar themes of recovery and discipleship. In fact, it seems that by comparing the seven miniletters to the selected representative churches in Asia Minor (Rev. 1:4, 11), a significant chiastic structuring emerges.

A Chiastic Understanding of Revelation 2–3[6]

A. (2:1–7) Church at Ephesus: an orthodox church in denial

  B. (2:8–11) Church at Smyrna: a faithful church suffering satanic abuse, told of short-term tribulation

    C. (2:12–17) Church at Pergamum: a compromising church, the majority standing firm but the minority in immoral practices

      D. (2:18–29) Church at Thyatira: a compromising church, persevering, but warned of great tribulation because of a lack of repentance (Note: The promises to overcomers and the charge, "He who has an ear, let him hear," reverse positions in the last four letters, likely implying a center-pivoting structure for the letters section.)

    C^1. (3:1–6) Church at Sardis: a compromising church, the majority incomplete and spiritually asleep, but some pure

  B^1. (3:7–13) Church at Philadelphia: a faithful church, suffering satanic abuse, told of protection from the worldwide hour of testing

A^1. (3:14–22) Church at Laodicea: a lukewarm church in denial

While it is not immediately clear what the wider significance of this inverted structure might be for an overall understanding of Revelation, two observations with great ramifications for recovery and discipleship can be made:

1. Recovery beyond denial and fully committed discipleship may entail great suffering, even while other professing believers are being pulled away into false teaching or immorality.
2. God allows tribulation in our lives (Acts 14:22), but he is fully able to protect his own from overwhelming suffering and to reward them for their faithfulness.

The Final Phase of the Great Commission

In Matthew 28:19–20 Christ commanded disciple making among "all the nations" by evangelism, baptizing, and teaching all the way until "the end of the age."[7] A little earlier he had also prophesied that "this gospel of the kingdom shall be preached in the whole world for a witness to all the nations, and then the end shall come" (Matt. 24:14).

Since the body of the Book of Revelation apparently deals largely with the end of the age,[8] the one passage that includes "gospel" (Rev. 14:6) would seem to be highly significant. That significance is also underlined by the far-reaching similarities between the extensive harvest imagery in Revelation 14 and the well-known parable of the wheat and tares (Matt. 13:36–43).[9]

These parallels become even more profound in the light of the inverted structure of Revelation 14–15. The following structural diagram seems to indicate that the final offer of the "eternal gospel" (14:6–7) is responded to by many from all nations, who are soon martyred and go victorious (through the blood of Christ; 12:11) into the presence of God (15:2–4). However, the two-sided harvest imagery (i.e., grain in 14:14–16, and grapes in vv. 17–20) reminds the reader that by no means will all respond positively, thereby avoiding the wrath of God (14:8–11).

The Inverted Structure of Revelation 14–15

A. (14:1–5) The Lamb on Mt. Zion (triumphant) with the 144,000, the "firstfruits" (of the harvest)

  B. (14:6–7) Final proclaiming of the eternal gospel to all nations because the hour of judgment is about to begin

    C. (14:8–11) Warning of God's wrath and judgment against those who follow Babylon the great and the Beast

      D. (14:12) Perseverance of saints (see 13:7) who keep the commandments of God and faith in Jesus (see 12:17)

E. (14:13) Blessing upon those who die in the Lord, for their works "follow" (see sixth blessing in 20:6)

D¹. (14:14–16) The (wheat) harvest of believers at the end of the age (see Matt. 13:36–43, parable of wheat and tares)

C¹. (14:17–20) Grape harvest/winepress of God's wrath (toward unbelievers)

B¹. (15:1–4) Those victorious (Greek *nikaō*; see 13:7) over the Beast, who have received the gospel from among all nations

A¹. (15:5–8) Sanctuary in heaven (see 13:6), preparing for the seven golden bowls full of the climactic wrath of God (i.e., the rest of harvest: "grapes of wrath"; see 14:17–20)

This structure reflects the completion of the Great Commission at the end of the age (Matt. 24:14; 28:19–20). All who are in the Lamb's book of life as disciples of the Lord (Rev. 13:8; 17:8) will be present and accounted for. They, like the 144,000, will "follow the Lamb (i.e., as disciples) wherever He goes" (14:4) from that point forward.

Beyond Recovery—Following Christ Forever

We must not overlook the glorious completion of the New Testament concept of recovery in Revelation! Because biblical recovery needs are anchored in the sinfulness of humanity, however, it cannot be said that recovery is over and done with until the sinfulness of humanity is no more.

That, of course, must be after the millennium[10] (one thousand years, mentioned only in 20:2–7), since people again rebel against the Lord at the end of that period (20:7–10). So, it is only the final judgment (20:11–15) and the emergence of the completely sin-free new heavens and earth (chaps. 21–22; see esp. 21:4–5, 27; 22:3) that once and for all rids redeemed mankind of the sin-darkened context in which recovery was needed.[11]

The many echoes of wording from the original creation and fall into sin (Gen. 1–3) leave the distinct impression that the eternal state (Rev. 21–22) is to be viewed as "Paradise Regained—*Permanently*" (with apologies to John Milton!). In the light of what has been seen throughout the New Testament, it will be a paradise characterized by the kind of discipleship longed for but not even possible in the present, limited, and sinful creation. And there will be no thought of recovery since everything having to do with the pain of the present created order will have long since "passed away" (21:4–5), forever and ever. Amen!

16

Pulling It All Together

Any attempt to compress the entire teaching of the New Testament on any subject into an at-a-glance form runs the decided risk of oversimplification. It is a risk worth taking, however, in order to provide a crisp means of grasping the general contours and the progress of the revelation of New Testament thought on the two rich topics of recovery and discipleship.

Table 16.1
Summarizing Recovery in the New Testament*

Gospels	Acts/Epistles	Revelation
Spiritual basis of recovery: Christ's person/work	Spiritual empowerment for recovery: Holy Spirit's New Covenant ministry	Emotional challenges to recovery: tribulation, abuse Ultimate outcome of recovery: eternal, wholeness

Gospels	Acts/Epistles	Revelation
Entering biblical recovery by faith	Progressing in biblical recovery through faith and disciplined obedience abuse	Continuing in recovery by overcoming Completing recovery eternally

*The authors have had the wonderful opportunity to team teach two courses on biblical and theological understanding and critique of recovery at Talbot School of Theology. Many of the angles presented in this book, including this chart, were born as questions, seminal ideas, or attempts to clearly communicate in those contexts where "What saith the Scriptures?" is the most basic ground rule.

Table 16.2
Discipleship in the New Testament

Gospels	Acts/Epistles	Revelation
Jesus as earthly Messiah/discipler	Jesus as heavenly high priest/object of discipleship	Jesus as coming King of Kings, along with followers
Disciples following Christ physically	Disciples committed to (i.e., following) Christ spiritually	Disciples committed through suffering, into Christ's presence
Disciples/followers	Church/saints believers/Christians	Overcomers/ repentant ones

There is also one further angle that will serve as the icing on the cake for *Disciplined Living*. In closing, we will momentarily move beyond the method of biblical theology and tie in recovery and discipleship with the systematic theology category of sanctification.[1] It is sincerely hoped that this last word (table 16.3) will help many readers wrap up recovery, discipleship, and sanctification all together into the package of maturing in Christ.

Table 16.3
Discipleship, Sanctification, and Recovery

Pre-Christian Status	Status in Christ	New Process Begun	Power Source	Classic Pitfall	Earthly Goal	Ultimate Goal
Unbeliever (volitionally)	Believer/ disciple	Growth in discipleship	Holy Spirit	Inconsistency as a disciple	Mature discipleship (and, for some, leadership)	Disciple like the teacher (forever!)
Sinner (theologically)	Justified	Growth in sanctification	Holy Spirit	Uneven sanctification	Holy, consistent lifestyle	Glorification (maximum sanctification)
Dysfunctional to some degree (emotionally/ relationally)	Recovering disciple	Progress in recovery	Holy Spirit	Regression in recovery	Healthy, consistent lifestyle/ relationships	Life beyond recovery forever

Notes

Introduction: *A Timely Warning*

1. The majority evangelical view is that Jude is the brother of James, the leader of the Jerusalem church (Acts 15:13; 21:18), and half brother of Jesus (Matt. 13:55), and that he was unbelieving (John 7:5) until sometime between the resurrection and ascension of Christ (Acts 1:9–11), since he is appropriately part of the prayerful group in the upper room between the ascension and Pentecost (Acts 1:13–14). See the similar discussion by Edwin A. Blum, "Jude," in *Expositor's Bible Commentary,* ed. Frank E. Gaebelein (Grand Rapids: Zondervan, 1981), 12:381.

2. This is the basic significance of the Greek term *mathētēs,* usually translated "disciple," which is used more than 250 times in the New Testament.

3. According to Donald Guthrie, *New Testament Introduction,* rev. ed. (Downers Grove, Ill.: InterVarsity Press, 1990), 908, the range of possible dates for the Epistle of Jude is A.D. 65 to 80. Blum, "Jude," 381, believes it could have been written as early as A.D. 60. Even the earliest dating would be some thirty years after the resurrection.

4. A. Boyd Luter, "James and Jude: A Recovery Profile," in *Life Recovery Bible,* eds. David Stoop and Stephen Arterburn (Wheaton, Ill.: Tyndale House, 1992), 1405.

5. Simply put, recovery is the comeback process from an unhealthy event, relationship, or behavior pattern that continues to impact a person's life in a negative way. Recovery issues are typical patterns in the life of a person who is resisting such emotional and spiritual recovery. The recovery movement is a loosely knit set of counseling centers and related ministries that apply Twelve Steps thinking in therapy programs. To be "in recovery" is to begin to try to solve the problems and alter the patterns that make a life dysfunctional, usually with the help of a counselor or other similar professional.

6. In the only two passages in which family members are named, Jude is listed fourth (Matt. 13:55) and third (Mark 6:3) among the sons. And, since "sisters" (Matt. 13:56; Mark 6:3) could have been interspersed in the order of children, Jude may well have been ten years (or more) younger than Jesus. If Joseph died when Jesus was, say, eighteen to twenty-two years old, Jude could easily have been as young as ten to fifteen, a very difficult and confusing stage

of life anyway. For a related discussion from the standpoint of James (Jude 1; Matt. 13:55), see A. Boyd Luter, "James, the Brother of Jesus," in *The Complete Who's Who of the Bible*, ed. Paul Gardner (Grand Rapids: Zondervan, 1995).

7. For a concise popular definition of recovery and the development of a biblical framework, see A. Boyd Luter, *Looking Back, Moving On: Applying Biblical Principles of Freedom to Your Life* (Colorado Springs: NavPress, 1993), 19.

For additional insight into the nature of discipleship, see Michael J. Wilkins, *Following the Master: Discipleship in the Footsteps of Jesus* (Grand Rapids: Zondervan, 1992); and A. Boyd Luter and Kathy McReynolds, *Women as Christ's Disciples: Biblical Models for Modern Discipleship* (Grand Rapids: Baker Books, forthcoming).

8. A. Boyd Luter and Kathy McReynolds, *Truthful Living: What Christianity Really Teaches about Recovery* (Grand Rapids: Baker Books, 1994).

9. A recent reflection of the tension was seen in a feature section of *Christianity Today*, 16 May 1994, that included the article "Psychobabble: A Guide for Perplexed Christians in an Age of Therapies," by Robert C. Roberts of Wheaton College and a sidebar interview with biblical counseling advocate David Powlison of Westminister Seminary (18–24).

10. Luter, *Looking Back, Moving On*, 18.

11. This is not to say that biblical proof-texts for certain views are not presented. It is to say that the way such texts are employed is often not in keeping with evangelical historical-grammatical contextual exegesis.

12. See chapter 11, table 11.1. This perspective is developed at length in chapter 3 of Luter and McReynolds, *Truthful Living*.

See also Stoop and Arterburn, *Life Recovery Bible*; Luter, *Looking Back, Moving On*; and McReynolds and Luter, "Recovering through Fully Biblical Recovery," *Christian Research Journal*, (spring 1993), 54.

13. Blum, "Jude," 389. See also Guthrie, *New Testament Introduction*, 909–12; and D. A. Carson, Douglas J. Moo, and Leon Morris, *An Introduction to the New Testament* (Grand Rapids: Zondervan, 1992), 462.

14. Jude 14–15 cites the Jewish pseudepigraphical Book of Enoch. This is not a problem for the evangelical doctrine of inspiration, since both Luke (Acts 17:28) and Paul (e.g., Titus 1:12) also cite extrabiblical writings.

15. The Greek work *eidos* (1 Thess. 5:22) has a range of meaning from the apparent "visible form" to an actual "kind" (of behavior).

16. This grave concern is developed in some depth in Luter and MeReynolds, *Truthful Living*, chapter 6.

17. Blum, "Jude," 395.

18. Blum, "Jude," 395, correctly sees three different groups of people to be dealt with in Jude 22–23.

Chapter 1: *Discipleship or Denial?*

1. Michael J. Wilkins, *The Concept of Disciple in Matthew's Gospel: As Reflected in the Use of the Term* Μαθητής (Leiden, The Netherlands: E. J. Brill, 1988).

2. Tim Stafford, "The Hidden Gospel of the Twelve Steps," *Christianity Today* (July 1991).

3. W. Bauer et al., *A Greek-English Lexicon of the New Testament and Other Christian Sources,* rev. ed. (Chicago: University of Chicago Press, 1979).

4. See the related discussion in chapter 8 of A. Boyd Luter and Kathy McReynolds, *Truthful Living: What Christianity Really Teaches about Recovery* (Grand Rapids: Baker, 1994).

5. D. A. Carson, Douglas J. Moo, and Leon Morris, *An Introduction to the New Testament* (Grand Rapids: Zondervan, 1992), 66–74.

6. A. Boyd Luter, "Matthew and Simon the Zealot: A Recovery Profile," in *Life Recovery Bible,* eds. David Stoop and Stephen Arterburn (Wheaton, Ill.: Tyndale House, 1992).

7. See the discussion of these Gentile women in Jesus' family tree in A. Boyd Luter, "Ruth" in A. Boyd Luter and Barry Davis, *The Books of God Behind the Seen: Expositions of Ruth and Esther, Expositor's Guides to the Historical Books* (Grand Rapids: Baker, 1995).

8. For a very useful discussion, with a conclusion for a dating in the 60s, see Carson, Moo, and Morris, *Introduction to the New Testament,* 76–79.

9. Though some liberals and a small number of evangelicals still date Matthew later than A.D. 70, the reasoning of John A. T. Robinson, in *Redating the New Testament* (Philadelphia: Fortress Press, 1976), seems to be holding sway. In essence, Robinson's central thesis is that, if an event as shaping as the destruction of Jerusalem (A.D. 70) had already occurred, it would be clearly discernible as a past-tense event in the New Testament, but it is not seen, so it probably hadn't occurred yet.

10. According to the standard New Testament Greek lexicon, (Bauer et al.) the meaning of the Greek word *arneomai,* which is normally translated "deny," is disown, renounce, or refuse (to acknowledge). Thus, there seems to be a strong overlap between the way the key term is used in the New Testament and the general recovery concept.

11. What was learned from this period of time has been previously shared in A. Boyd Luter, *Looking Back, Moving On: Applying Biblical Principles of Freedom to Your Life* (Colorado Springs: NavPress, 1993).

12. Josh McDowell speaks to this deficient view in his perceptively titled book, *More Than a Carpenter* (San Bernadino, Calif.: Here's Life Publishers, 1981).

13. A good place for the serious student to start would be Michael J. Wilkins, "Matthew: Examples with a Commission," in *Following the Master: Discipleship in the Footsteps of Jesus* (Grand Rapids: Zondervan, 1992), 174–93.

14. For further insight into all the passages in Matthew in this section, see representative evangelical commentaries such as D. A. Carson, "Matthew," in *Expositor's Bible Commentary*, ed. Frank E. Gaebelein (Grand Rapids: Zondervan, 1984); J. Knox Chamblin, "Matthew," in *Evangelical Commentary on the Bible*, ed. Walter A. Elwell (Grand Rapids: Baker, 1989); and Richard T. France, *Matthew*, Tyndale New Testament Commentaries (Grand Rapids: Eerdmans, 1985).

15. Sadly, Matthew 10:24–25a, and its apparent counterpart in Luke 6:40, have both often been abused by ignoring their immediate contexts. The difficulty of discipleship is ignored by failing to recognize that the true Teacher/Master we follow is often called "the ruler of the demons" (Matt. 12:24), or something similar, as 10:25b makes clear. In Luke 6, the danger of following the wrong kind of teacher is emphasized in verses 39–40 as having "potentially disastrous consequences" (Thomas R. Schreiner, "Luke," in *Evangelical Commentary*, ed. Elwell, 814).

16. See the in-depth discussion of Mary as a disciple in chapter 3 of A. Boyd Luter and Kathy McReynolds, *Women as Christ's Disciples: Biblical Models for Modern Discipleship* (Grand Rapids: Baker, forthcoming).

17. See the complementary insights concerning the women disciples at the foot of the cross in Luter and McReynolds, *Women as Christ's Disciples*, chapters 2 and 5.

18. See the discussion in chapter 5 of this book. For more in-depth development of the Great Commission, see A. Boyd Luter, "Discipleship and the Church," *Bibliotheca Sacra* (July–September 1980), 167–73; A. Boyd Luter, *A New Testament Theology of Discipling* (Ann Arbor, Mich.: University Microfilms/Th.D. diss., Dallas Theological Seminary, 1985); A. Boyd Luter, "Great Commission," in *Anchor Bible Dictionary*, ed. David Noel Freedman (Garden City, N.Y.: Doubleday, 1992); and Luter and McReynolds, "Unexpected Disciples and the Great Commission," chapter 2 in *Women as Christ's Disciples*.

19. For a compact treatment of what is known about this disciple, see A. Boyd Luter, "Joseph of Arimathea," in *The Complete Who's Who of the Bible*, ed. Paul Gardner (Grand Rapids: Zondervan, 1995).

Chapter 2: *The Reality of Suffering and Recovery*

1. C. S. Lewis, *The Problem of Pain* (New York: Macmillan, 1962), 90.

2. Lewis, *Problem of Pain*, 90.

3. Lewis, *Problem of Pain*, 93.

4. C. S. Lewis, *A Grief Observed* (London: Bantam Books, 1963), 41–42. The reader should note that the recent popular movie *Shadowlands* did largely communicate accurately the sense of pain and grief surrounding Joy

Gresham's death. However, the extent of Lewis's theological wrestling was not completely conveyed.

5. George MacDonald, Unspoken Sermons. First Series, microfiche.

6. While there are some legitimate questions about the reliability of Irenaeus's claim and early church tradition, their testimonies have been generally accepted by most scholars.

7. Walter W. Wessel, *The Book of Mark*, vol. 8 of *The Expositor's Bible Commentary*, ed. Frank E. Gaebelein (Grand Rapids: Zondervan, 1984), 608–11; Craig S. Keener, *The IVP Bible Background Commentary: New Testament* (Downers Grove, Ill.: InterVarsity Press, 1993), 132–34; D. E. Nineham, *Saint Mark* (Baltimore: Penguin Books, 1963), 29–34.

8. Mark's Gospel, as with all the writings of the New Testament, was written to a specific people for a specific purpose. But this in no way diminishes God's Word from speaking, in context, to all believers in all generations.

9. Tacitus, quoted by Everett Ferguson, *Backgrounds of Early Christianity* (Grand Rapids: Eerdmans, 1987), 472.

10. Ferguson, *Backgrounds of Early Christianity*, 474–75.

11. Gaebelein, ed., *Expositor's Bible Commentary*, 610.

12. See Mark 8:14–21; 9:14–32 for other examples of the disciples' lack of faith and understanding.

13. Max Lucado, *No Wonder They Call Him Savior* (Portland, Ore.: Multnomah, 1986), 95.

Chapter 3: *Calling All Outcasts and Sinners!*

1. It is clear that, while Jesus closely associated with sinners, he neither participated in nor condoned their sin.

2. Craig S. Keener, *The IVP Bible Background Commentary: New Testament* (Downers Grove, Ill.: InterVarsity Press, 1993), 187.

3. See Keener, *IVP Commentary*, 185–86; Robert Maddox, *The Purpose of Luke–Acts* (Edinburgh: T & T Clark Ltd., 1982), 12–15; Walter L. Liefeld, "The Gospel of Luke," in *The Expositor's Bible Commentary*, ed. Frank E. Gaebelein (Grand Rapids: Zondervan, 1984), 8:797–815.

4. See chapter 5 for a more detailed discussion on Luke's purpose in the Book of Acts.

5. Leon Morris, *Tyndale New Testament Commentaries: Luke*, rev. ed. (Grand Rapids: Eerdmans, 1988), 39.

6. There is a detailed account of the events surrounding the birth of Christ in Luke 1–2. No other Gospel writer chronicles his birth so completely as Luke.

7. Frederick Buechner, *The Hungering Dark* (New York: Seabury, 1981), 13–14.

8. This, of course, excludes participation in sinful activities. He did not possess a sinful nature.

9. For a more complete discussion on the work of the Holy Spirit in the church, see chapter 5.

Chapter 4: *That You May Believe . . .*

1. H. E. Dana, *The New Testament World*, 3d ed., (Nashville: Broadman, 1937), 201–56. Daily life in the Jewish home was considerably different than in the non-Jewish home. There was generally more structure and order within the family unit (149–56).

For more background on Gentile society and culture in the first century, see also Everett Ferguson, *Backgrounds of Early Christianity* (Grand Rapids: Eerdmans, 1987), 36–110.

2. Dana, *New Testament World*, 231.

3. Dana, *New Testament World*, 231. See also Ferguson, *Early Christianity*, 99. He discusses how easy it was to get a divorce in the first century.

4. The Synoptics are the other three Gospels: Matthew, Mark, and Luke.

5. There is some question as to whether *believe* is in the present subjunctive (that you may continue to believe) or in the aorist subjunctive (that you may believe) in the original manuscript. The latter has more manuscript evidence, while the former version is older. See Merrill C. Tenney, "Gospel of John," in *The Expositor's Bible Commentary*, ed. Frank E. Gaebelein (Grand Rapids: Zondervan, 1984), 9:197. It is not clear whether John was writing to strengthen those who were already believers or to evangelize unbelievers. Nevertheless, the Gospel can certainly address the needs of both.

6. Tenney, "Gospel of John," 9:12.

7. Tenney, "Gospel of John," 9:13.

8. However, a bad relationship with our parents will oftentimes distort our concept of God. We may project onto the Father the shortcomings and failures of our parents. But we have learned from John that times of questioning and faltering are a common, valid part of the true believer's experience.

Chapter 5: *Recovering Disciples, Building Blocks of the Church*

1. This approach to outlining Acts is developed in D. A. Carson, Douglas J. Moo, and Leon Morris, *An Introduction to the New Testament* (Grand Rapids: Zondervan, 1992), 181–85.

2. See the in-depth discussion of denial in the Gospel of Matthew, including Peter's focal episode, in chapter 1.

3. This approach to outlining Acts is developed in William H. Baker, "Acts," in *Evangelical Commentary on the Bible*, ed. Walter A. Elwell (Grand Rapids: Baker, 1989), 885. A more complex variation on this approach is utilized by

Stanley D. Toussaint, "Acts," in *Bible Knowledge Commentary: New Testament,* eds. John F. Walvoord and Roy B. Zuck (Wheaton: Victor, 1983), 352–53.

4. For an in-depth discussion of Dorcas and her ministry to the widows in Joppa, see "Dorcas: A Model Disciple," chapter 8 in A. Boyd Luter and Kathy McReynolds, *Women as Christ's Disciples: Biblical Models for Modern Discipleship* (Grand Rapids: Baker, forthcoming).

5. For a related discussion of John Mark from a recovery perspective, see A. Boyd Luter, *Looking Back, Moving On: Applying Biblical Principles of Freedom to Your Life* (Colorado Springs: NavPress, 1993), 83–85. It should also be noted here that, over time, Paul radically changes for the better his perception of Mark (e.g., see 2 Tim. 4:11).

6. For a discussion of the significance of the mention of this woman in Acts 16, see "Partners in the Gospel: The Women in the Church at Philippi," chapter 11 in Luter and McReynolds, *Women as Christ's Disciples.*

7. Most commentators simply ignore (or dodge) the question of whether this woman was converted or not. But, if she had not been, the demon (or demons) would undoubtedly have returned with a vengeance to reclaim her (see Matt. 12:43–45), which apparently did not occur (Acts 16:19–22).

8. See the helpful introductory discussions of the authorship of Acts in Baker, "Acts," in *Evangelical Commentary,* ed. Elwell, 883; and Carson, Moo, and Morris, *Introduction to the New Testament,* 185–90.

9. This issue of whether growing believers can have recovery issues is discussed at some length in the introductory chapter of Luter, *Looking Back, Moving On.*

10. Various reasons have been proposed for the seemingly strange absence of this terminology. For a helpful discussion, see Michael J. Wilkins, *Following the Master: Discipleship in the Footsteps of Jesus* (Grand Rapids: Zondervan, 1992), 283–89.

11. That conclusion only makes sense since the Great Commission in Matthew commands disciple making until "the end of the age" (28:19–20). This line of reasoning was originally developed in A. Boyd Luter, "Discipleship and the Church," *Bibliotheca Sacra* (July–September 1980), 167–73.

12. For two complementary comprehensive studies of the New Testament usage, see Richard D. Calenberg, "The New Testament Doctrine of Discipleship" (Th.D. diss., Grace Theological Seminary, 1983); and A. Boyd Luter, *A New Testament Theology of Discipling* (Ann Arbor, Mich.: University Microfilms/Th.D. diss., Dallas Theological Seminary, 1985).

13. See the extensive discussion of the key discipleship principles in Matthew 10 in chapter 1.

14. This phenomenon is also discussed with its specific significance for Dorcas in chapter 8 of Luter and McReynolds, *Women as Christ's Disciples.*

15. Wilkins, *Following the Master*, 249; and Wilkins, "Disciples," in *Dictionary of Jesus and the Gospels*, eds. Joel B. Green, Scot McKnight, and I. Howard Marshall (Downers Grove, Ill.: InterVarsity Press, 1992), 178.

16. Evangelical scholars are not in agreement as to whether Matthew was one of Luke's sources. However, there is something of a consensus that either Matthew or much of Matthew's source material was available to Luke in writing his two-volume work: the Third Gospel and Acts. See the varying brief, but helpful, discussions in Thomas R. Schreiner, "Luke," in *Evangelical Commentary on the Bible*, ed. Elwell, 802–3; John A. Martin, "Luke," in *Bible Knowledge Commentary*, eds. Walvoord and Zuck, (Wheaton, Ill.: Victor, 1983), 199, 201; and Carson, Moo, and Morris, *Introduction to the New Testament*, 118–21.

17. The final phase of the Great Commission, reflecting the completion of the Lord's global prediction in Matthew 24:14 and the process mandated in 28:19–20, will be discussed in the concluding chapter of this book.

18. This same unrealistic and damaging perspective is critiqued in appendix A of Luter, *Looking Back, Moving On*, 169–71.

19. A related discussion of a biblical basis for a support group approach, as well as a critique of how the evangelical Recovery Movement often misuses such methodology, is found in chapter 10 of A. Boyd Luter and Kathy McReynolds, *Truthful Living: What Christianity Really Teaches about Recovery* (Grand Rapids: Baker, 1994).

Chapter 6: *Spiritual Freedom and Recovery*

1. Martin Luther, quoted by James M. Kittelson, "The Accidental Revolutionary," *Christian History* 11 (34):12.

2. For an extended discussion on this view, see Everett F. Harrison, "Romans," in *Expositor's Bible Commentary*, ed. Frank E. Gaebelein (Grand Rapids: Zondervan, 1976), 10:5–6.

3. Wolfgang Wiefel, "The Jewish Community in Ancient Rome and the Origins of Roman Christianity," in *The Romans Debate*, ed. Karl Donfried (Peabody, Mass.: Hendrickson Publishing, 1991), 95–96.

4. James Montgomery Boice, "Galatians," in *Expositor's Bible Commentary*, ed. Gaebelein, 10:410. See also his extended discussion on the background of the Galatian churches, 10:409–20.

5. Walt Russell, "The Apostle Paul's View of the 'Sin Nature'/'New Nature' Struggle," in *Christian Perspectives on Being Human: A Multidisciplinary Approach to Integration*, eds. J. P. Moreland and David M. Ciocchi (Grand Rapids: Baker, 1993), 208.

6. For example, see Herman Ridderbos, *Paul: An Outline of His Theology*, trans. John R. DeWitt (Grand Rapids: Eerdmans, 1975), 57–68; Charles R.

Smith, "Two Natures—or One? An Attempt at Theological Clarification," *The Voice* (July–August 1983), 19–21; John M. G. Barclay, *Obeying the Truth: Paul's Ethics in Galatians* (Minneapolis: Fortress Press, 1988); Douglas J. Moo, "Israel and Paul in Romans 7:7–12," *New Testament Studies* 32 (1986): 122–35; Mark W. Karlberg, "Israel's History Personified: Romans 7:7–13 in Relation to Paul's Teaching on the 'Old Man.'" *Trinity Journal* 7 (1986): 64–74.

7. Russell, "Apostle Paul's View," 209.

8. Ridderbos, *Paul,* 66–67.

9. Russell, "Apostle Paul's View," 211. For an extended discussion on the usages of *flesh* and *Spirit* in the Pauline epistles, see Russell's entire article, 207–27.

10. Moo, "Israel and Paul," 124–25, 129.

11. Russell, "Apostle Paul's View," 217.

12. See Russell's redemptive-historical interpretation of Galatians 5:16–18, "Apostle Paul's View," 216–17.

13. Russell, "Apostle Paul's View," 218.

Chapter 7: *Confronting Chronic Immaturity*

1. D. A. Carson, Douglas J. Moo, and Leon Morris, *An Introduction to the New Testament* (Grand Rapids: Zondervan, 1992), 263.

2. Excellent compact discussions of the history of Corinth and the transition from the "old Corinth" to the "new Corinth" can be found in James A. Davis, "1–2 Corinthians," in *Evangelical Commentary on the Bible,* ed. Walter A. Elwell (Grand Rapids: Baker, 1989), 958–59; and Carson, Moo, and Morris, *Introduction to the New Testament,* 263.

3. It is highly likely that Paul spent the bulk of the three months mentioned in Acts 20:3 in Corinth and wrote Romans from there in about A.D. 55 or 56. The mention of former coworkers from Corinth such as Prisca and Aquila (Rom. 16:3–4) supports such a view (Royce G. Gruenler, "Romans," in *Evangelical Commentary,* ed. Elwell, 924).

4. A recent broader evangelical source that develops this background in detail is B. W. Winter, *Are Paul and Philo among the Sophists? A Hellenistic Jewish and a Christian Response to a First Century Movement* (Ph.D. diss., Macquarie University, 1988).

5. If the chronology of Paul's ministry in Carson, Moo, and Morris, *Introduction to the New Testament,* is reasonably accurate, all the events in this listing would have taken up no more than six or seven years.

6. This is clearly the basic organizing principle of the outline of 1 Corinthians in Davis, "1–2 Corinthians," 963.

7. E.g., Gordon D. Fee, *The First Epistle to the Corinthians,* New International Commentary on the New Testament (Grand Rapids: Eerdmans, 1987), 16–17.

8. It is not within the purpose of this presentation to debate the theories of whether 2 Corinthians 8–9 or 10–13 were originally separate letters. Such usually liberal hypotheses are skillfully answered by Carson, Moo, and Morris, *Introduction to the New Testament*, 267–77.

9. Adapted from the outline in A. Boyd Luter, "2 Corinthians," study notes, in *Life Recovery Bible*, eds. David Stoop and Stephen Arterburn (Wheaton, Ill.: Tyndale House, 1992), 1281.

10. Adapted from Craig A. Blomberg, "The Structure of 2 Corinthians 1–7," *Criswell Theological Review* 4 (fall 1989), 3–20.

11. See the in-depth exposition (including this problem) of 2 Corinthians 10–13 in D. A. Carson, *From Triumphalism to Maturity* (Grand Rapids: Baker, 1984).

12. For a significant, and largely unique, treatment of this central passage on spiritual gifts, see D. A. Carson, *Showing the Spirit: A Theological Exposition of 1 Corinthians 12–14* (Grand Rapids: Baker, 1987). Though the writer cannot agree with Carson at all points, his perspective and argumentation is consistently challenging and thought provoking.

13. See chapter 11 for a discussion of maturity related to leadership in 1–2 Timothy and Titus.

14. See the related discussion of 2 Corinthians 12:9–10 in A. Boyd Luter, *Looking Back, Moving On: Applying Biblical Principles of Freedom to Your Life* (Colorado Springs: NavPress, 1993), 106–11.

Chapter 8: *Recovering the New Self*

1. A baby buster is anyone born between 1963 and 1977.

2. Andres Tapia, "Reaching the First Post-Christian Generation," *Christianity Today* (12 September 1994), 18–19. Used with permission.

3. Tapia, "Post-Christian Generation," 20–22.

4. For a more detailed discussion on the similarities and differences between Ephesians and Colossians, see Curtis Vaughan, "Colossians," in *The Expositor's Bible Commentary*, ed. Frank E. Gaebelein (Grand Rapids: Zondervan, 1978), 11:168–69.

5. Vaughan, "Colossians," 166. Colossians and Philemon were likely written at the same time. See chapter 9 for a discussion on the origin of these two epistles.

6. For a more in-depth discussion on the background of Colossae and the purpose for Paul's letter to them, see Donald Guthrie, *New Testament Introduction*, rev. ed. (Downers Grove, Ill.: InterVarsity Press, 1990), 564–84.

7. See Guthrie, *New Testament Introduction*, 496–540, for an extended discussion on the background, purpose, and destination of Ephesians.

8. A. Skevington Wood, "Ephesians," in *Expositor's Bible Commentary*, ed. Gaebelein, 11:26.

9. Francis Foulkes, *The Epistle of Paul to the Ephesians*, Tyndale New Testament Commentaries (London: Tyndale House, 1963), 65.

10. Wood, "Ephesians," 59.

11. For instance, the apostle John describes the new life in Christ as "abiding in" or "being in" Jesus (John 15; 1 John).

12. Donald Guthrie, *New Testament Theology* (Downers Grove, Ill.: InterVarsity Press, 1981), 647.

13. Guthrie, *New Testament Theology*, 658.

Chapter 9: *Twin Case Studies in Intervention*

1. The concept of intervention is typically used in recovery circles to speak of a person or persons stepping in to attempt to stop the reeling-out-of-control lifestyle of a person either dependent on alcohol or drugs or notably abusive toward a loved one. As will be seen, from a biblical perspective, this recovery angle on intervention is too narrow (and often too late).

2. It has been standard practice for commentaries to pair Philemon together with Colossians, apparently because Philemon lived in Colossae and was a member of the Colossian church. Some modern evangelical examples of such an approach are William Hendricksen, *Exposition of Colossians and Philemon*, New Testament Commentary (Grand Rapids: Baker, 1964); Robert G. Gromacki, *Stand Perfect in Wisdom: An Exposition of Colossians and Philemon* (Grand Rapids: Baker, 1981); Ralph P. Martin, *Colossians and Philemon*, New Century Bible (Grand Rapids: Eerdmans, 1981); Peter T. O'Brien, *Colossians, Philemon*, Word Biblical Commentary (Waco: Word, 1982); and Robert Wall, *Colossians and Philemon*, IVP New Testament Commentaries (Downers Grove, Ill.: InterVarsity Press, 1993).

3. It is comparatively rare for a commentary volume in a series to treat these two letters together. Two notable older exceptions are Marvin R. Vincent, *A Critical and Exegetical Commentary on the Epistles to the Philippians and to Philemon*, International Critical Commentary (Edinburgh: T & T Clark, 1897); and Jacobus J. Muller, *The Epistles of Paul to the Philippians and to Philemon*, New International Commentary on the New Testament (Grand Rapids: Eerdmans, 1955).

4. Among the better evangelical introductions to how biblical chiasmus works are H. Van Parunak, "Some Axioms for Literary Architecture," *Semeia* 8 (1983), 1–16; and Ronald E. Man, "The Value of Chiasm for New Testament Interpretation," *Bibliotheca Sacra* (1984).

5. An important older study that took on that erroneous outlook has recently been republished as Nils Lund, *Chiasm in the New Testament* (Peabody, Mass.: Hendrickson, 1992).

6. Two of the more helpful of these are John W. Welch, ed., *Chiasmus in Antiquity* (Gerstenberg, Germany: Hildesheim, 1981); and Craig L. Blomberg, "The Structure of 2 Corinthians 1–7," *Criswell Theological Review* (1989), 3–20.

7. The fact that almost no Old Testament quotations or clear allusions appear in either book strongly supports that contention. Also, the apparent lack of the minimum number to comprise a Jewish synagogue in Philippi points in that direction. See John B. Polhill, *Acts*, New American Commentary (Nashville: Broadman, 1992), 348.

8. This A B C B¹ A¹ structure is only a slightly more sophisticated arrangement than the most basic A B A¹ or A B B¹ A¹ inverted parallelism (Parunak, "Literary Architecture," 8). The possibility that the perceived chiasm is merely coincidental would be much greater, though, if Philemon were not as closely related to Philippians in circumstances and themes, since a strong case can be made that Philippians is, in fact, constructed as a grand chiasm (see note 11 below).

9. A prominent evangelical example of such an understanding is Robert H. Mounce, "Philippians," in *Wycliffe Bible Commentary*, eds. Everett F. Harrison and Robert Pfeiffer (Chicago: Moody, 1962), 1320.

10. The nature of the intervention in Philippians is developed in A. Boyd Luter, "Partners in the Gospel: The Role of Women in Philippians and the Church at Philippi," *Journal of the Evangelical Theological Society* (forthcoming), and chapter 11 of A. Boyd Luter and Kathy McReynolds, *Women as Christ's Disciples: Biblical Models for Modern Discipleship* (Grand Rapids: Baker, forthcoming).

11. The evidence for and extent of the parallelism in this suggested structure was initially developed in depth in A. Boyd Luter and Michelle V. Lee, "Philippians as Chiasmus: Key to the Structure, Unity and Theme Questions," *New Testament Studies* (1995), 89–101. Both of the studies cited in note 10 (Luter, "Partners in the Gospel"; Luter and McReynolds, *Women as Christ's Disciples,* chapter 11) also discuss the textual basis and implications of this inverted parallel structure. It is also noteworthy that a similar, but somewhat less complex, chiastic structuring of Philippians has recently been published by Charles H. Talbert, "Philippians," in *Mercer One-Volume Commentary on the Bible*, ed. Watson E. Mills (Macon, Ga.: Mercer University Press, 1994).

12. Of the thirteen uses of *sunergos* in the New Testament, twelve are in Paul's letters. Yet he never uses the word to speak specifically of anyone other than a close, and highly committed, disciple.

13. This is in keeping with the cultural way that Greeks looked down on their slaves/servants during this era. R. W. Paschal Jr., "Service," in *Dictionary of Jesus and the Gospels*, eds. Joel B. Green, Scot McKnight, and I. Howard Marshall (Downers Grove, Ill.: InterVarsity Press, 1992), 748.

14. D. A. Carson, Douglas J. Moo, and Leon Morris, *An Introduction to the New Testament* (Grand Rapids: Zondervan, 1992), 388, present a plausible reconstruction of the situation in Philemon against the backdrop of Roman slavery.

15. It is not at all unlikely that the original difference between the two ladies was quite petty, given that absolutely nothing is said by Paul in Philippians about its precipitating cause. Nor is there any sense about who was right, only that *both* were wrong in the way they handled the situation (i.e., actually refusing to face their own individual responsibility).

16. The most obvious reason for the churchwide impact would seem to be the almost unique prominence of women in the foundation and earlier development of the church at Philippi, including Euodia and Syntyche (Phil. 4:2–3), among all the churches seen in the New Testament. See Luter, "Partners in the Gospel"; and Luter and McReynolds, *Women as Christ's Disciples*, chapter 11.

17. While it is virtually a principle of even most evangelical recovery counselors that people will not wholeheartedly face their problem(s) until they hit bottom, that should not have to be the case with Christians, who have the Holy Spirit within to convict them of sin related to their fearful (and, very often, prideful) denial and help them face the situation, no matter how difficult, with "love, joy, peace" and, yes, "self-control" (Gal. 5:22–23).

18. For an in-depth discussion of the unity factor in the context of Ephesians 4:1–16 and its immense implications for recovery, see chapter 1 in A. Boyd Luter and Kathy McReynolds, *Truthful Living: What Christianity Really Teaches about Recovery* (Grand Rapids: Baker Books, 1994).

19. Peter T. O'Brien, *Commentary on Philippians*, New International Greek Testament Commentary (Grand Rapids: Eerdmans, 1991), 477–78.

20. Carson, Moo, and Morris, *Introduction to the New Testament*, 388–89; and Ralph P. Martin, *Philippians*, New Century Bible (Grand Rapids: Eerdmans, 1980), 152.

Chapter 10: *Be Ready for Recovery*

1. For further discussion on the length of time Paul spent in Thessalonica, see Warren W. Wiersbe, *Be Ready* (Wheaton, Ill.: Victor Books, 1982), 10–13; D. Edmond Hiebert, *The Thessalonian Epistles: A Call to Readiness* (Chicago: Moody, 1971), 16–17.

2. Craig S. Keener, *The IVP Bible Background Commentary: New Testament* (Downers Grove, Ill.: InterVarsity Press, 1993), 371–72.

3. Richard N. Longnecker, "Acts," in *The Expositor's Bible Commentary*, ed. Frank E. Gaebelein (Grand Rapids: Zondervan, 1981), 9:470.

4. Wiersbe, *Be Ready*, 18.

5. W. E. Vine, *The Expanded Vine's Expository Dictionary of New Testament Words* (Minneapolis: Bethany House, 1984), 562–63.

6. Romans 8:28 and Philippians 4:4–7 are also often quoted to people who are suffering.

Chapter 11: *Building on Recovery and Discipleship*

1. Frequently this first inviting recovery comfort zone will be a support group. Under the umbrella of a safe, nonjudgmental environment, even a church-based support group can stagnate. Rather than supporting a person as he or she strives for progress in recovery and Christian growth, they support someone as having a right to be a bitter victim who does little more than vent or whine. See the discussion of God's intention that the church be the primary supportive group for Christians with deep hurts and other needs in chapter 5. See also the related discussion of support groups from a scriptural perspective in A. Boyd Luter and Kathy McReynolds, *Truthful Living: What Christianity Really Teaches about Recovery* (Grand Rapids: Baker, 1994).

2. Relatively little is known about Titus, but he hardly emerges as a flamboyant, Peter-like personality. Rather, he appears to be a steady, trustworthy disciple whom Paul could count on in difficult situations, such as dealing with the Corinthian church (2 Cor. 7–8).

3. William H. Baker, "Acts," in *Evangelical Commentary on the Bible,* ed. Walter A. Elwell (Grand Rapids: Baker, 1989), 920.

4. The apparent possibility of death is alluded to in Philippians 1:19–24, but the wording is so vague that there is no way to determine how serious the threat of death might have been.

5. The likely chronology of the latter stages of the apostle's public ministry is discussed helpfully, but briefly, in George W. Knight III, "1–2 Timothy/-Titus," in *Evangelical Commentary,* ed. Elwell, 1099–1100.

6. The title "Pastoral Epistles" has been in use since the early 1700s and has been defended recently as legitimate by evangelicals such as Knight, "1–2 Timothy/Titus," 1098; and D. A. Carson, Douglas J. Moo, and Leon Morris, *An Introduction to the New Testament* (Grand Rapids: Zondervan, 1992), 359.

7. Other reservations about the title are expressed by Gordon D. Fee, *1 and 2 Timothy, Titus,* Good News Commentary (San Francisco: Harper and Row, 1984).

8. For a helpful popular treatment of what is known of Timothy's life, see William J. Petersen, *The Discipling of Timothy* (Wheaton, Ill.: Victor Books, 1980). Current study related to Timothy as a disciple, with muted recovery ramifications, is found in chapter 12 of A. Boyd Luter and Kathy McReynolds, *Women as Christ's Disciples: Biblical Models for Modern Discipleship* (Grand Rapids: Baker, forthcoming).

9. For a parallel perspective on contemporary American society, see Boyd Luter, *Looking Back, Moving On: Applying Biblical Principles of Freedom to Your Life* (Colorado Springs: NavPress, 1993), 19–20.

10. Helpful discussions of these qualifications can be found in Knight, "1–2 Timothy/Titus." See also Knight's much longer treatment, *The Pastoral Epistles*, New International Greek Testament Commentary (Grand Rapids: Eerdmans, 1993). Fee, *1 and 2 Timothy, Titus*, is quite helpful but should be read cautiously, with his feminist agenda in mind.

11. Note the apparent interchangeability of *elder* with *overseer* (or *bishop*) in Acts 20:17, 28 and Titus 1:5, 7.

Chapter 12: *Tandem Explorations of Trust Issues*

1. Through church history, the diverse non-Pauline letters of the New Testament usually have been called the "Catholic Epistles" or the "General Epistles." A less common, but plausible, alternative title is the "Jewish Christian Epistles."

See the excellent compact survey of the extent of influence of the Pauline authorship of Hebrews view in D. A. Carson, Douglas J. Moo, and Leon Morris, *An Introduction to the New Testament* (Grand Rapids: Zondervan, 1992), 394–96.

2. The mention of "twelve tribes" and the use of the Greek term *diaspora* in James 1:1 certainly implies the concept of the Jewish "Diaspora" (i.e., Jews living outside of Palestine), but is no more nailed down in terms of location.

3. This understanding is certainly enhanced by the fact that the title "To the Hebrews" was already attached at the earliest points at which it shows up in church history (Carson, Moo, and Morris, *Introduction to the New Testament*, 401).

4. For a compact biographical treatment of James, see A. Boyd Luter, "James, the Brother of Jesus," in *The Complete Who's Who of the Bible*, ed. Paul Gardner (Grand Rapids: Zondervan, 1995).

5. See A. Boyd Luter, "A Recovery Profile: James and Jude," in *Life Recovery Bible*, eds. David Stoop and Stephen Arterburn (Wheaton, Ill.: Tyndale House, 1992), 1405; and the parallel discussion about Jude in the introduction to this book.

6. The most likely explanation for the otherwise strange silence about Joseph in the Gospel narratives of Jesus' public ministry is that he was already dead. For a discussion of this question, see A. Boyd Luter, "Joseph, the Husband of Mary," in *Who's Who of the Bible*, ed. Gardner.

Assuming Joseph's death, Jesus, as the oldest son, would have become the functional head of the household. In addition, he almost certainly took over the running of Joseph's carpentry business (being called "the carpenter's son" in Matt. 13:55 and "the carpenter" in Mark 6:3), with the younger brothers, like James and Jude, working under him.

7. Carson, Moo, and Morris, *Introduction to the New Testament,* 409.

8. See also a very plausible alternative outlining of James in D. J. Moo, "James," in *Evangelical Commentary on the Bible,* ed. Walter A. Elwell (Grand Rapids: Baker, 1989), 1153.

9. For more insight on specific recovery factors, see A. Boyd Luter, "Hebrews," study notes, in *Life Recovery Bible,* eds. Stoop and Arterburn, 1379–97.

10. Carson, Moo, and Morris, *Introduction to the New Testament,* 392.

11. Thanks to former student Professor Victor Rhee of Talbot School of Theology for very helpful interaction on the thought and structure of the Epistle to the Hebrews. Professor Rhee is completing "The Concept of Faith in Hebrews," Ph.D. diss., Dallas Theological Seminary.

12. See the more conventional alternative outline in Robert S. Rayburn, "Hebrews," in *Evangelical Commentary,* ed. Elwell, 1131.

13. Of the sixteen uses of *faith* (Greek *pistis*) in James, eleven are located in 2:14–26. All three occurrences of *to believe* (or *trust*) (Greek *pisteuō*) are in 2:14–26.

14. The relationship between faith and works in James 2:14–26 was most troubling to Martin Luther during the Reformation Era and reerupted as a center of controversy most recently in the so-called "Lordship salvation" debate.

15. Longstanding attempts to portray James and Paul as being contradictory on faith and works completely blow out of proportion what is nothing more than different, but complementary, emphases.

16. Of the thirty-two uses of *faith* in Hebrews, twenty-eight are found in 10:19–12:29 (and twenty-four of those are in chapter 11, the well-known "faith chapter").

Chapter 13: *Perspectives of a Recovered Disciple*

1. This particular passage has been understood in various ways. For an in-depth discussion on the various interpretations, see D. A. Carson, "Matthew," in *Expositor's Bible Commentary,* ed. Frank E. Gaebelein (Grand Rapids: Zondervan, 1984), 8:367–75.

2. Herbert Lockyer, *All the Apostles of the Bible* (Grand Rapids: Zondervan, 1972), 130.

3. Philip Yancey, *Disappointment with God* (Grand Rapids: Zondervan, 1988), 151–52.

4. Lockyer, *All the Apostles,* 150.

5. For a more in-depth discussion on the recipients and purpose of 1 and 2 Peter, see Edwin A. Blum, "1 and 2 Peter," in *Expositor's Bible Commentary,* ed. Gaebelein, 12:212–13, 262–63.

6. Warren Wiersbe, *Be Hopeful* (Wheaton: Victor, 1983), 13–14.

Chapter 14: *The Gnostic Error and Recovery*

1. Glenn W. Barker, "1, 2, 3 John," in *Expositor's Bible Commentary*, ed. Frank E. Gaebelein (Grand Rapids: Zondervan, 1981), 12:293–98.

2. Curtis Vaughan, *Bible Study Commentary: 1, 2, 3 John* (Grand Rapids: Zondervan, 1970), 8–10; Craig S. Keener, *The IVP Bible Background Commentary: New Testament* (Downers Grove, Ill.: InterVarsity Press, 1993), 734–36; B. F. Westcott, *The Epistles of St. John* (Grand Rapids: Eerdmans, 1966), xxxiii–xxxviii.

3. Barker, "1, 2, 3 John," 293.

4. Henry Cloud and John Townsend, *False Assumptions* (Grand Rapids: Zondervan, 1994), 126.

5. For a more in-depth discussion on the nature of human beings and the effects of sin as it relates to recovery issues, see A. Boyd Luter and Kathy McReynolds, *Truthful Living: What Christianity Really Teaches about Recovery* (Grand Rapids: Baker, 1994).

6. Another example of this is the apostle Paul's warning to the Colossian believers about certain philosophies and practices, which seemed to be a seminal form of Gnosticism (Col. 2:6–23).

7. Vaughan, *1, 2, 3 John*, 8–10. For a more in-depth discussion on the development of Gnosticism, see Everett Ferguson, *Backgrounds of Early Christianity* (Grand Rapids: Eerdmans, 1987), 240–49.

Chapter 15: *Concluding the Great Commission and Recovery*

1. For a presentation of the key recovery themes in Revelation, see A. Boyd Luter, "Revelation," study notes, in *Life Recovery Bible*, eds. David Stoop and Stephen Arterburn (Wheaton, Ill.: Tyndale House, 1992), 1449–72. For a compact treatment of the eschatology (teaching on last things) of recovery, see "Biblical Recovery over the Long Haul," chapter 11 in A. Boyd Luter and Kathy McReynolds, *Truthful Living: What Christianity Really Teaches about Recovery* (Grand Rapids: Baker, 1994).

2. Not only is it placed last in the order of New Testament books, Revelation also gives more detailed biblical information about the end of the age and the transition to eternity future than any other biblical book. An interesting, though hardly certain, canonical perspective on Revelation is argued by Robert W. Wall, *Revelation*, New International Biblical Commentary (Peabody, Mass: Hendrickson, 1991), 29–32.

3. Despite some apparent evidence to the contrary, the most likely conclusion on the authorship of Revelation is still that it was written by the apostle John. See D. A. Carson, Douglas J. Moo, and Leon Morris, *An Introduction to the New Testament* (Grand Rapids: Zondervan, 1992), 468–73.

4. The most likely position is still that John is "the beloved disciple." See Gary Burge, "John," in *Evangelical Commentary on the Bible*, ed. Walter A. Elwell (Grand Rapids: Baker, 1989), 841–42.

5. Interestingly, of the forty-five uses of the Greek term *thlipsis*, usually translated "tribulation" in the New Testament, only five to seven unequivocally deal with the end of the age. The other thirty-eight to forty deal with suffering during the course of the age, while the five to seven speak of unparalleled suffering in the context preceding Christ's second coming.

6. A less precise chiastic structuring of the seven letters in Revelation 2–3 has been noted by Wall, *Revelation*, 68–69, citing Leon Morris, *The Revelation of St. John*, Tyndale New Testament Commentaries (Grand Rapids: Eerdmans, 1969), 57–58.

7. See the earlier discussions on the Great Commission in chapters 1 (on Matthew) and 5 (on Acts).

8. Carson, Moo, and Morris, *Introduction to the New Testament*, 483, say "Revelation is about eschatology, not history."

9. For example, both Alan Johnson, "Revelation," in *Expositor's Bible Commentary*, ed. Frank E. Gaebelein (Grand Rapids: Zondervan, 1981), 12:543; and Walter Elwell, "Revelation," in *Evangelical Commentary*, 1219, toy with the possibility that the harvest in Revelation 14:14–16 might be related to the fields white unto harvest (Matt. 9:37–38; John 4:35) imagery for an evangelistic harvest, then reject the idea in favor of a harvest of judgment. Neither seems to have seriously considered how close the wording is to the wheat and tares in Matthew 13:36–43, which portays a two-sided (i.e., salvation and judgment) harvest.

10. While the authors are premillennialists, it is not the purpose of this volume to debate systematic eschatological positions. Rather, it is to lay out biblical theological themes significant to the interweaving of the overall New Testament teaching on discipleship and recovery.

11. See especially the brief discussion of recovery themes related to the new heavens and earth in Revelation 21–22 in chapter 11 of Luter and McReynolds, *Truthful Living*.

Chapter 16: *Pulling It All Together*

1. In a number of the chapters in this book, sanctification has already emerged as a parallel concept to both long-term biblical recovery and discipleship. Though the authors have largely been responsible for exploring the linkage between recovery and discipleship up to this point, I acknowledge my debt in earlier research on the basic theological equivalence of discipleship and sanctification to Richard D. Calenberg, "The New Testament Doctrine of Discipleship" (Th.D. diss., Grace Theological Seminary, 1983).

Selected Bibliography

Since no theology of recovery related to discipleship has ever previously been published, there are no resources that closely parallel the present volume. The following modest listing includes evangelical works of some real significance for the fields of recovery (from a strong biblical perspective) and discipleship, as well as the chosen methodology of New Testament biblical theology and the integration of psychology and theology. The vast majority have been produced since 1980.

Calenberg, Richard D. "The New Testament Doctrine of Discipleship." Th.D. diss., Grace Theological Seminary, 1983.

Carson, D. A., Douglas J. Moo, and Leon Morris. *An Introduction to the New Testament.* Grand Rapids: Zondervan, 1992.

Carter, John, and Bruce Narramore. *The Integration of Psychology and Theology.* Grand Rapids: Zondervan, 1979.

Davis, John Jefferson. *Foundations of Evangelical Theology.* Grand Rapids: Baker, 1984.

Elwell, Walter A., ed. *Baker Encyclopedia of the Bible.* 2 vols. Grand Rapids: Baker, 1988.

———. *Evangelical Commentary on the Bible.* Grand Rapids: Baker, 1989.

———. *Evangelical Dictionary of Theology.* Grand Rapids: Baker, 1984.

Green, Joel. B., Scott McKnight, and I. Howard Marshall, eds. *Dictionary of Jesus and the Gospels.* Downers Grove, Ill.: InterVarsity Press, 1992.

Guthrie, Donald. *New Testament Introduction,* rev. ed. Downers Grove, Ill.: InterVarsity Press, 1990.

———. *New Testament Theology.* Downers Grove, Ill.: InterVarsity Press, 1981.

Hart, Archibald. *Me, Myself and I.* Ann Arbor, Mich.: Servant Publications, 1992.

Hawthorne, Gerald F., Ralph P. Martin, and Daniel Reid, eds. *Dictionary of Paul and His Letters.* Downers Grove, Ill.: InterVarsity Press, 1993.

Ladd, George E. *A Theology of the New Testament.* Grand Rapids: Eerdmans, 1974.

Luter, A. Boyd, Jr. "Discipleship and the Church." *Bibliotheca Sacra* (July–September 1980), 167–73.

———. "Great Commission." In *Anchor Bible Dictionary.* Ed. by David Noel Freedman. Vol. 2. Garden City, N.Y.: Doubleday, 1992.

———. *Looking Back, Moving On: Applying Biblical Principles of Freedom to Your Life.* Colorado Springs: NavPress, 1993.

———. *A New Testament Theology of Discipling.* Dallas: Dallas Theological Seminary; Ann Arbor, Mich.: University Microfilms, 1985.

Luter, A. Boyd, Jr., and Kathy McReynolds. "Recovering through Fully Biblical Recovery." *Christian Research Journal* (spring 1993).

———. *Truthful Living: What Christianity Really Teaches about Recovery.* Grand Rapids: Baker, 1994.

———. *Women as Christ's Disciples: Biblical Models for Modern Discipleship.* Grand Rapids: Baker, forthcoming.

Ridderbos, Herman. *An Outline of Paul's Theology.* Trans. by John Richard DeWitt. Grand Rapids: Eerdmans, 1974.

Ryrie, Charles C. *A Biblical Theology of the New Testament.* Chicago: Moody Press, 1963.

Stafford, Tim. "The Hidden Gospel of the Twelve Steps." *Christianity Today,* July 1991.

———. "The Therapeutic Revolution." *Christianity Today,* August 1993.

Stoop, David, and Stephen Arterburn, eds. *Life Recovery Bible.* Wheaton, Ill.: Tyndale House, 1992.

Vos, Geerhardus. *Biblical Theology.* Grand Rapids: Eerdmans, 1948.

Wilkins, Michael J. *The Concept of Disciple in Matthew's Gospel: As Reflected in the Use of the Term* Μαθητής. Leiden, The Netherlands: E. J. Brill, 1988.

———. *Following the Master: Discipleship in the Footsteps of Jesus.* Grand Rapids: Zondervan, 1992.

Subject Index

Scripture Index

Genesis

1–3—180
12—160
12:2—22
12:3—21
17:13—95

1 Samuel

16:7—104

Isaiah

53:3—55

Jeremiah

17:9—20

Matthew

Book of—21
1:1—21
1:3—22
1:5—22
1:6—22
4:18–20—156
7:13–14—21
9:9—21
10:1–4—19
10:2—156
10:3—21
10:24–25—81
10:24–39—20
12:46–50—14
13:36–43—179, 180
13:55—148
13:55–57—13
14:28—154
14:28–31—156
15:15—157
15:18—155
15:26–27—22

16:16—154, 156
16:18—77, 83
16:18–19—156
16:21–22—56
16:22—154, 162
17:1–8—156
18:21—157
20:25–28—144
24:14—179, 180
26:31–35—19
26:33–35—157
26:35—154
26:36–46—156
26:58—157
26:58–75—19
26:69–75—78, 157
26:74—154
27:3–5—37
27:35–50—14
27:55–56—14
28:17—74
28:19—19, 22, 83
28:19–20—82, 83, 84, 179, 180
28:20—83

Mark

1:16–18—156
1:23–25—43
1:29—155
1:32–34—43
2:1–12—43
2:14–17—21
3:1–6—43
3:10–11—43
3:16—156
3:20–21—41
3:31–35—41
3:35—41
4:35–41—43

4:38—43
5:8—51
5:24–34—37
5:37—156
7:1–23—44
7:6–7—44
7:14–15—44
7:18—44
7:20–23—44
8:29—156
8:31—41
8:34–36—41
9:2–8—156
10:28—154
10:29–31—41
10:30—42
10:32–34—41
10:35–45—42
10:43–44—42
10:45—42
11–16—38
13:34—157
14:12–31—44
14:31—44
14:32–41—44
14:33–42—156
14:37—41
14:50—45
14:54—45, 157
14:66–72—37, 45, 157
16:7—37, 45

Luke

1:1–4—81
1:3—51
1:4—52
2:10—53
2:14—53
2:32—53
2:42–48—13–14

208

About the Authors

Boyd Luter (B.S., Mississippi State University; Th.M., Ph.D., Dallas Theological Seminary) is adjunct professor of biblical studies at Golden Gate Baptist Theological Seminary: Southern California Campus. He has written *Looking Back, Moving On* and co-authored *God Behind the Seen: Expositions of the Books of Ruth and Esther,* as well as contributing to such biblical resource works as the *Evangelical Commentary on the Bible, Anchor Bible Dictionary,* and *The Complete Who's Who of the Bible.*

Kathy McReynolds (B.A., Biola University; M.A., Talbot School of Theology) contributed to the *Life Recovery Bible* (Tyndale House) and *Who's Who in the Bible* (Harper/Collins, 1994). She has team-taught a theology of recovery course with Dr. Luter at Talbot School of Theology. Together they have written *Truthful Living: What Christianity Really Teaches about Recovery.*